W9-BLS-480

The Yoga Facelift

The Yoga
Facelift

MARIE-VÉRONIQUE NADEAU

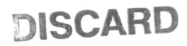

First published in 2007 by Conari Press, an imprint of Red Wheel/Weiser, LLC

With offices at:
500 Third Street, Suite 230
San Francisco, CA 94107
www.redwheelweiser.com

ISBN-10: 1-57324-278-0

ISBN-13: 978-1-57324-278-3

Library of Congress Cataloging-in-Publication Data

Nadeau, Marie-Véronique.

The yoga facelift / Marie-Véronique Nadeau. p. cm.

ISBN 1-57324-278-0 (alk. paper)

1. Facial exercises.
2. Hatha yoga.
3. Beauty, Personal. I. Title.

RA778.N25 2007

646.7'26--dc22

2006027002

Cover and book design by Yoshie Matsumoto

Typeset in ITC Officina Sans, Aldus, and FF Scala

Photographs by Joshua Abeyta

Printed in Hong Kong

SS

10 9 8 7 6 5 4 3 2 1

Contents

Introduction

None of us were born yesterday (or we wouldn't be reading this)—yet why is it we are constantly browbeaten into believing we should look as though we were? We're told we should erase all the evidence of our life experience—the love and laughter, grief and pain, any and everything pertaining to our emotional testament. Needless to say, this program is not about promoting this dreadfully mistaken notion. Having lived life to its fullest, I see the implicit beauty that stems from experience as something far more attractive than the faux youth look achieved today via dubious makeover procedures.

Proudly brandishing the badge of my "advanced" age (fifty-eight and soon to be a grandmother for the first time, for those who are curious), I can sincerely say that I've never felt more vivacious or self-assured in my life. Naturally I am bursting to share my discoveries in the field of skin care with those who know in their hearts that inner beauty won't be coaxed out by the swipe of a surgeon's blade or the puncture of a Botox syringe. I'm all for embellishing my facial portrait, but not necessarily that way.

Proper nutrition, therapeutic skin products, and attitude modification are the triple engines of my alternative beauty program. But before we discuss those, please let me introduce the subject addressed by the book you are holding: exercise.

Nowadays we have all kinds of exercise programs that give our torsos, backs, buttocks, everything from the shoulder blades down to the toes, a workout. We have Pilates, Nautilus machines, and calisthenics, to mention just a few. But as far as I know nobody is paying much attention to the most hard-working set of muscles of our entire body—those operating under that wrinkled wasteland from the neck up! Why is it that we religiously maintain our pecs, biceps, and posteriors, but from the collarbone up we resign ourselves to wrinkles and sags? What you probably don't realize is that the very strain of exercising all those lower limb and lumbar regions are making your face and neck sag and wrinkle much faster, making you look much older than your years. It seems to me that there is a real paradox at work here—we are trying so hard to look good in places we can always cover up, yet we are neglecting the one part that for most of us is always naked. This is clearly a lopsided allocation of energy and resources.

The intuitive reader might suggest that I am advocating a lazy person's design for living here. And about time, I say. The Yoga Facelift is the perfect exercise program for those of you who, like me, are addicted to the fine art of relaxation. Not only can you stop apologizing and/or feeling embarrassed about your sloth, but you also now have something to be sanctimonious about the next time your pals try to drag you to some smelly gym. You simply tell them, "Exercise the Yoga Facelift way! You can be a couch potato and still remain a hot tomato." Once they've had some time to think it over, they'll probably thank you for releasing them from treadmill bondage.

To my surprise, what began as a light-hearted attempt to bring a little fun into the grim business of working out soon blossomed into a program that was not only enjoyable, but also actually produced discernible results. Adults of all ages in my classes were feeling and looking better, giving me an implicit vote of confidence to proceed with my alternative beauty program. One friend now claims that she owes her success rate on the dating circuit to three conditions: native charm (25 percent), exercise (25 percent), and Marie-Véronique skin therapy (50 percent).

Microcurrent vs. Exercise

Recently many people have been asking me what I think about microcurrent, the "new technology" (it's really neither new nor much of a technology—it's actually been around in one form or another almost since the invention of the light bulb) in which electrical stimulation contracts muscles to tone and lift the face. Clearly, my exercise program is based on a similar idea—muscles lengthen over time, imparting to the face the classic sag of aging. Contracting facial muscles, via exercise or some other way, shortens them, so sagging is reduced and the face overall takes on a toned and more youthful appearance. This seems to beg the question: if the outcome with microcurrent is the same as with exercise, why bother with laborious calisthenics when I can lie back and be zapped into youth and beauty? I believe there are differences between the two rejuvenation techniques that are worth considering.

First of all, as with any technology involving electrical current, microcurrent is an unknown quantity. Though it is described as noninvasive, we don't really know what the long-term effects might be. When you can easily contract your own muscles, why would you subject yourself to bursts of current, no matter how low-level (microcurrent devices are defined as using less than 500 microamperes)? I also have aesthetic reservations; listen to this description of the procedure: "the operator . . . uses probes to perform what is known as muscle reeducation. Through a series of assertive scooping and contouring movements the operator can lengthen or shorten muscles on demand." Frankly, I wouldn't trust my one and only face to some operator whose training and sensibility I can only guess at. I believe the *only* person capable of performing such delicate operations on one's face is one's self. That is why in *The Yoga Facelift* you learn techniques for reshaping your face that rely on *your* intuition and knowledge.

There is also the question of cost—the national average for each microcurrent treatment is $110, with a suggested series of seven to twelve treatments. I firmly believe that you will get more pleasing results, and be safer and healthier in the long run, for the price of this book.

It's been my experience that alternative practices work better than conventional medical techniques or faddish cosmetic treatments, and the reason is simple. We have only to remember that the body is very wise, and given the least bit of encouragement it can do wonders to heal and help itself. As Jacques Cousteau once said, "Nature is a great protector." He was talking about areas of the ocean greatly affected by pollution. When left alone they recovered with a rapidity that was almost miraculous. The same thing applies, dear students, to your face. Try it and see.

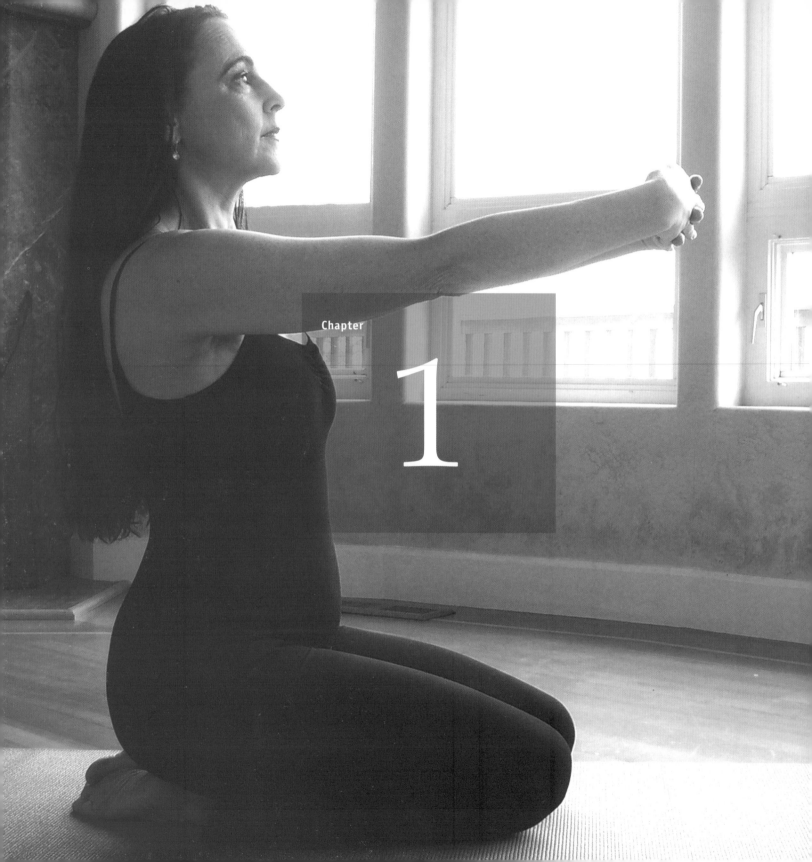

How the Yoga Facelift Works

The rationale behind the Yoga Facelift is simple: the face is the gateway to the soul, but the stresses and strains of daily living often prevent us from putting our best face forward. When we were told as kids that if we made funny faces they might stick that way, there was a grain of truth hiding behind the teasing. Facial expressions that reflect worry, unhappiness, and anger have a way of becoming permanent. The good news is that we are not stuck with what we see in the mirror—if we don't like what we see, *we can change it.*

▶ The Physical Aspect

There are a number of ways we can effect change. First of all, from a purely physical stand-point, exercises do a lot to counteract the effects of time and gravity. Over time our muscles lengthen as gravity pulls ever downward, causing the sagging we start to see everywhere in our faces; eyes start to droop, foreheads and cheeks sag, and jowls start to form until it's almost like watching a snowman melt in slow motion. Exercising shortens muscles, and so we end up with tighter, firmer faces as we tone the musculature underneath. This method of addressing sagging is far superior to plastic surgery, the other option, because it actually im-proves your appearance over time. Plastic surgery is at best a temporary fix, and sometimes it isn't the fix you were hoping for. A conventional facelift simply stretches skin over the same old flabby muscles, and gravity starts to work immediately to undo the lift. The other, more serious problem associated with cosmetic surgery is that conventional treatments often give people a very unnatural, blank, or stretched look. Wiping all the character from a person's face is the most profound form of identity theft I can imagine.

▶ The Spiritual Aspect

Yoga exercises are as mentally and spiritually beneficial as they are physically beneficial. In stark contrast to surgery, yoga exercises create change from within by bringing the mind and body into harmony. Yoga facelift exercises bring all parts of ourselves into harmony, including that part of our body that acts a conduit to the world outside—the face. The face is our in-terface (an apt word) with the world, the means by which we receive and convey a great deal of information. It's not surprising then that the face tends to be the big giveaway to hidden turmoil—our faces can, and often do, reflect disharmonies in ourselves. That means we may be conveying messages to the outside world that we do not intend and are not even feeling, simply because we have fallen into habits of expression as we fall into habits of speech and thinking. Awareness is the first step towards changing that. As Anaïs Nin put it: "We don't see the world as it is, but as we are."

Changing What We See

Nin's observation is certainly true enough, but this interface starts to get really complicated when we ask the question: so what does the world (that is, other people) see when it sees us? The answer is complex (oh, these big brains of ours) because two dynamics are intertwined; others see you according to their own program, but also according to your program—that is, they are seeing you as *they* are, but also as *you* are. To make it even more dizzying, this "as you are" isn't usually the real you; rather, it's a marriage of your projection onto them with their projection onto you. No wonder most marriages end in divorce.

Hopefully behind all the smoke and mirrors a glimmer of the real you lurks, prepared to peek out. In any case, the goal of the Yoga Facelift is to bring into better harmony all those disparate elements that fragment and trouble our souls. It might be helpful to think of the world out there as our mirror, but along with that vision comes the understanding that what we need to do to change our reflection is to change *ourselves*, not the mirror.

To make a long journey short, when we become aware of what we are doing with our faces, as we are aware of what we are doing with our bodies, we find that with conscious effort, diligent application, and some time, we *can* effect change. Like sculptor's clay, the flesh can be shaped, molded, and remodeled with massage, exercise, and attitude. Change may happen primarily from the inside out, but it's quite astonishing how much we can do to help it along by also working from the outside in.

How Long Does It Take?

At first, a complete set of exercises takes about one hour to do. As you become more accomplished and once your muscles get into shape, you can get by with a maintenance program of ten to fifteen minutes a day. Eventually you might need to do only a Quick Lift set every other day or so.

Another advantage of these exercises is you don't need to set aside time to do them. Just pick out the exercises that are most useful to you, then practice them whenever you have a few minutes. For example, if you work in front of the computer, take a break by doing stretches or "palming" and other eye exercises.

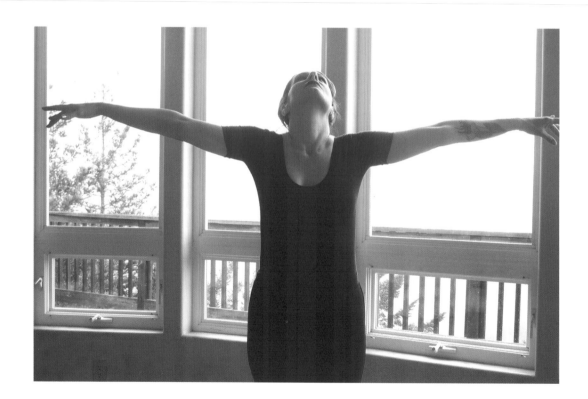

Who Can Do the Yoga Facelift?

The beauty of the Yoga Facelift is that anyone can do it almost anywhere, anytime. Whether you are in a wheelchair, ninety years old, or a just a busy person always on the go, you can benefit from the exercises in this book. What's more, you don't need special clothing, bouncy balls, spongey mats, or any kind of equipment. All you need is a mirror, this book, and a willingness to try.

A Note to Botox Patients

I should note here that there is one group of people who won't be able to do these exercises, at least at first—those who have had recent Botox work. Of course, you are the folks who need it the most. Muscle atrophy follows muscle paralysis, so if you've had Botox treatments, you should start your exercise programs as soon as possible after having the procedure done. And even before the rest of your face responds you will still be able to benefit from the neck and jawline exercises, as well as those that work with any other area not directly affected by Botox. It is very important for you to get in the habit of exercising your muscles instead of immobilizing them. Once your face starts collapsing plastic surgery might be your *only* option. The adage "if you don't use it, you lose it" really applies to the muscles of your face.

How to Use This Book

This book offers exercises for all levels, from beginning to advanced. They are numbered (1) for beginners, (2) for intermediate students, and (3) for advanced students based on their level of difficulty. This categorization is of course very subjective, and it's based principally on what my students tell me they find easy, somewhat easy, or difficult.

You might find some of the beginner exercises rather difficult at first, because you are using muscles that you are not accustomed to having control over—in many cases you are working with muscles you didn't even know you had (this is especially true of the eye area). My advice is to just stick with them, and the exercises you hate at first may become your favorites after some practice. But some exercises, even those I've put in the advanced category, might seem easy to you! Everyone is different.

The exercises themselves are divided into groups that target different areas. For example, the exercises for eyes, forehead, and neck are arranged so that you can select from each group at least one exercise that will benefit you. After you've tried all the exercises, incorporate those that seem most useful into your own exercise routine. I include my own favorite exercise routine as an example. You will get more out of the exercise program by choosing those exercises that address those areas that are of concern to you and concentrating on them. For example, I once worked with a middle-aged student whose facial muscles were so firm and toned that if it weren't for her droopy neck you'd put her age at twenty years younger than she actually was. We devised a program that addressed her one problem area, and now she often has to assure people that she really is a grandmother in her late fifties.

Last but not least, please bear in mind that facial workouts are quite different from other workouts. Being consistent will bring better results than undertaking marathon sessions that leave you exhausted. As you can see from the photos, you can do these exercises just about anywhere, so you don't need to set aside a time and place to do them. Spend just five or ten minutes *every day*—while you're sitting in traffic, while you're cooking dinner, or while you're watching TV—doing some of the exercises you've selected, and after a very short time you will see marvelous results. Usually people start to see changes in as little as two to three weeks, and certainly by the end of two to three months you will start seeing significant changes.

▶ The Quick Lift

Once you have faithfully practiced your exercises for three months or so (it could be as little as a month, it just depends on how quickly you see results), then you are ready for a maintenance program. The Quick Lift requires only two or three minutes of your time each day and is marvelous all-over exercise that will keep your toned face in great shape. Folks on the maintenance program can do the Quick Lift five days a week, and a longer, ten- to fifteen-minute program one day a week. Choose one out of the seven days week to rest.

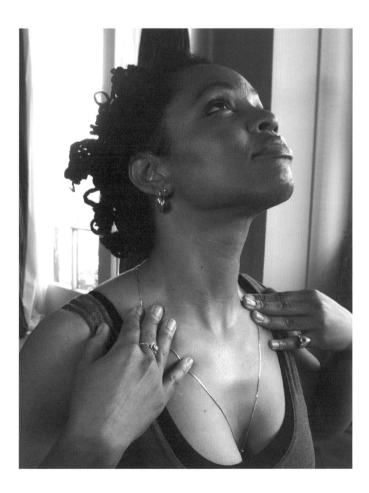

Exercise Hints

1. **Isolate**. At first, look in a mirror when you are doing some of these exercises to make sure you are not making lines elsewhere in your face when you are doing them. Keep the muscles that are not involved in a particular exercise relaxed. After some practice you will be able to feel what you are doing and you won't need your mirror. For example, if you are one of those people who concentrates by drawing her eyebrows together, pay attention to that area, and try to keep it relaxed. Be aware of the areas where you are holding tension, or where you are contracting muscles.

2. **Breathe!** Maintaining a breathing pattern makes exercising much more effective. When you contract a muscle, inhale, hold your breath while you are holding a contraction, and exhale as you release.

3. **Visualize.** Picture the expression you want to convey (happy, relaxed) and what muscles you want to call into play to create it. The facial muscles illustration of at the end of this chapter will help you visualize what is happening underneath the skin as you do the exercises.

4. **Modify.** With a little modification, all of the exercises in this book can be done by people whose mobility is limited. For example, the exercises that begin in a standing position can just as easily begin in a seated position.

5. **Have fun.** As the guru says, if you're not having fun, you're not being serious. I want you to be serious in the sense of having fun, but I don't think you should take this or any other self-help program too seriously. To paraphrase our guru, if you're not having fun, you're not going to get the results you want.

Now we're ready for the exercises. Remember, have fun and keep smiling!

A Note to Scowlers

Brow furrowers or frowners are earnest folk (you know who you are) who convey seriousness by contracting their brows together. A good first exercise that will help you get in the spirit of the Yoga Facelift is to think about other ways to convey gravitas or to convince others you are really paying attention. Try nodding, or murmuring "uh huh" or "nyuh uh" or whatever they say in your neck of the woods at regular intervals, or tapping your finger against your chin or scratching your head. You may look silly, but at least it beats the hell out of Botox.

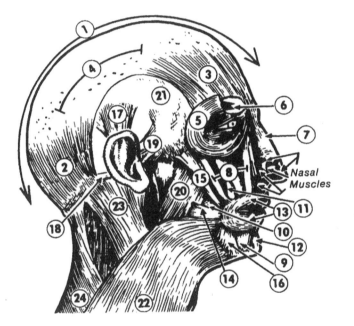

Nasal
Muscles

Muscles of the Face and Neck

1. Epicranius or occipito frontalis covers the top of the skull and consists of two parts: the occipitalis and the frontalis

2. Occipitalis—the back part of the epicranius

3. Frontalis—the front part of the epicranius

4. The aponeurosis—a tendon that holds together the occipitalis and the frontalis

5. Obicularis oculi—surrounds the eye socket

6. Corrugator—the Botox scowl muscle

7. Procerus—lies across the bridge of the nose

8. Quadratus labii superioris—three parts; raises and draws back the upper lip and nostrils

9. Quadratus labii inferioris—controls the lower lip

10. Buccinator—compresses the cheeks

11. Caninus—raises the lips, as in a snarl

12. Mentalis—in the tip of the chin—raises the lower lip

13. Orbicularis oris—surrounds the lips

14. Risorius—draws back lips, as in grinning

15. Zygomaticus—elevates the upper lip

16. Triangularis—draws down the corners of the mouth

17, 18, and 19. Muscles of the ear

20 and 21. Masseter and temporalis—the chewing muscles

22. Platysma—depresses the lower jaw and lower lip

23. Sterno-cleido-mastoid—rotates the head and bends the neck

24. Trapezius—back of the neck—rotates the shoulder blades and controls swinging of the arms

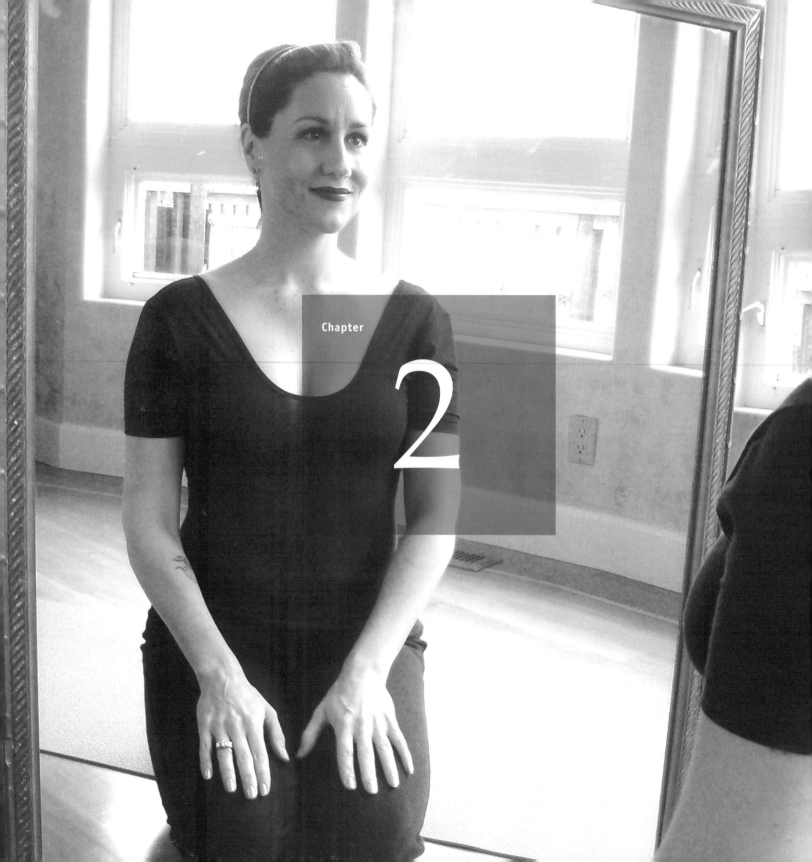

Chapter

2

Getting Started

You should always start your exercise routine with a simple warm up—it can be as easy as just doing one breathing and one stretching exercise. It's amazing how five minutes just breathing and stretching can alter your frame of mind and brighten your whole day.

▶ **Breathers**

Always start your exercise routine with breathing, bearing in mind that maintaining a smooth breathing pattern makes exercising much more effective. When you contract a muscle, inhale, hold your breath while you are holding a contraction, and exhale as you release.

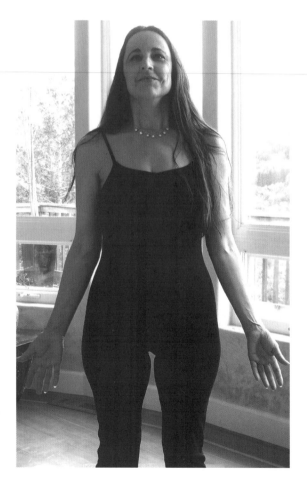

Stand and Breathe, Pose 1

Stand and Breathe (1)

Stand with your feet slightly apart. Inhale, lift your rib cage, draw in your abdominal muscles, relax your shoulders (Pose 1). Hold for a count of ten. Exhale, letting out all the air, then exhale even more deeply, pushing all the stale air out of your diaphragm, for a count of ten.

Do this three times.

Bend and Breathe (1)

Stand with your feet slightly apart. Inhale. As you bend over from the waist exhale, and lift your arms up as high as you can towards the ceiling in back of you (Pose 1). Hold for a count of five, then come up on your inhalation, lifting your arms towards the sky or the ceiling (Pose 2).

Hold for a count of ten. Repeat two times.

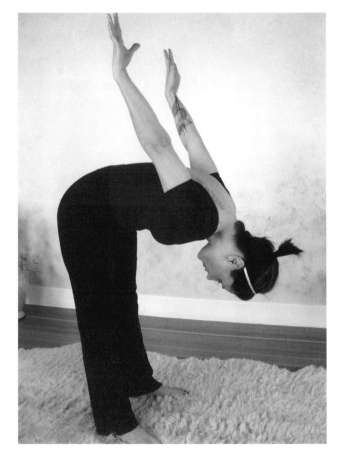

Bend and Breathe, Pose 1

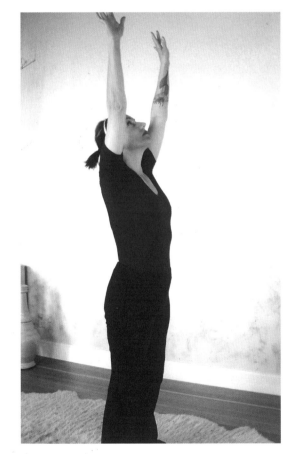

Bend and Breathe, Pose 2

Spine Stretcher/Energizer (1)

Stand with your feet slightly apart, knees slightly bent. Relax your shoulders, relax your neck, relax your arms. Now bend over at the waist and let your arms dangle while you stay completely relaxed (Pose 1). It doesn't matter if you hands touch the floor. Don't reach—just relax forward and let gravity gently stretch the spine.

As you come up, straighten your legs and come up onto the balls of your feet, breathe in, and stretch your arms towards the ceiling as high as you can go (Pose 2).

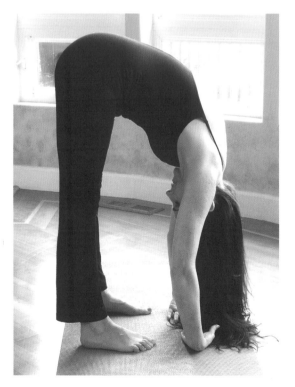

Spine Stretcher/Energizer, Pose 1

Hold for a good twenty seconds, really stretching—you can always stretch higher than you think you can. Exhale forcefully, with a "whoosh" of breath, then release your arms and let them dangle towards the floor as you bend over from the waist again.

Repeat ten times.

On the final time, come back up from your last waist bend to stand quietly, breathing and really feeling your beautiful straight spine. Notice the energy radiating to all parts of the rest of your body from your spine. Thank your spine for supporting you in all your endeavors.

This exercise is a wonderful warm up and energizer. If you have time for only one exercise, do this one. Or any time during the day when you are feeling tired, just take a break and do this spine stretcher—you'll feel instantly energized, particularly if you remember to really breathe.

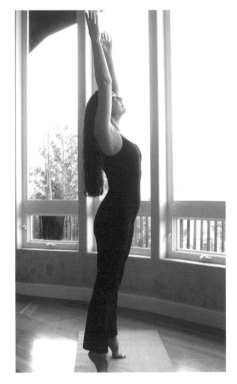

Spine Stretcher/Energizer, Pose 2

The Turtle (2)

Stand or sit upright. Pull your chin in towards your chest, like a turtle pulling into its shell (Pose 1).
Now slowly bring your head forward and upward, as if the turtle were poking its head out of its shell
(Pose 2). Hold for a count of five. Pull your chin in and down, like a turtle retracting his head into
his shell.

Repeat two times.

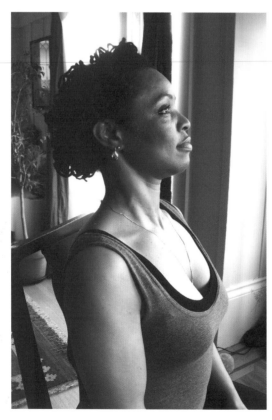

The Turtle, Pose 1

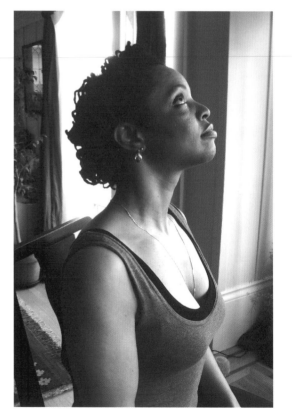

The Turtle, Pose 2

Arms and Shoulders (3)

This exercise helps to draw the shoulders back and, incidentally, works to tighten sagging upper arms.

Stand with your legs about a foot apart, knees relaxed. Raise your arms so they are horizontal to each side of your body (Pose 1). Now raise your shoulders to meet your ears. Then move your arms behind you, palms facing up, until they almost meet in back; relax your shoulders (Pose 2).

With gentle movements, move your arms towards each other, so that the thumbs almost, but not quite, touch in back. Do this motion 100 times. The trick here is to keep your arms lifted in back as high as you can while keeping your shoulders relaxed. The higher your arms, the greater the tightening action. After the last time, release and shake out your arms.

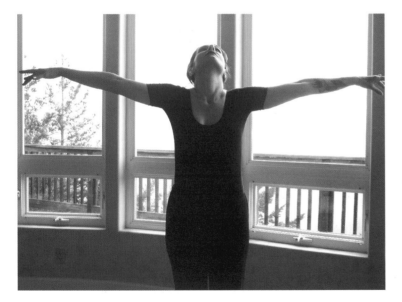

Arms and Shoulders, Pose 1

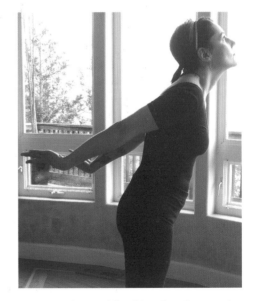

Arms and Shoulders, Pose 2

Cow Face (3)

The Cow Face is an excellent yoga posture that really stretches the spine. Raise your right arm vertically so that your upper arm is next to your right ear and then bend it at the elbow so your hand is resting on your upper right side of your back, as if you were patting yourself on the back. Reach your left arm around your left side and up towards the left side of your back (Pose 1). Reach up with your left hand towards the fingertips of right hand, while your right hand is stretching towards the fingertips of your left hand. Now stretch your hands together until your fingertips touch. The goal is to get your two sets of fingertips to touch each other in the middle of your back (Pose 2). If you can't get your fingertips to touch don't worry, just get as close as you can and still be comfortable. The more you do this, the more of a stretch you will be able to get. Soon you will find that your fingertips will touch without effort.

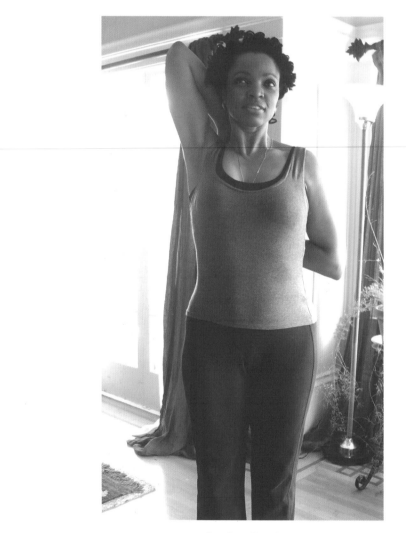

Cow Face, Pose 1

Relax your shoulders, hold your chin up, hold for a count of ten. Release your arms and take a deep breath.

Repeat two more times.

Now do the same for the other side. This time, raise your left arm up next to your left ear and reach down the back with your left hand, while you reach around with your right hand. Hold for ten, then relax your arms and take a deep breath.

Repeat twice.

By now we're standing tall and straight without effort. So let's have a look at our posture.

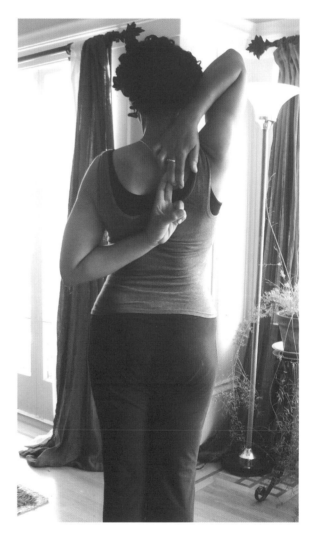

Cow Face, Pose 2

▶ Posture

Be aware of your posture as you walk. Keep your pelvis tucked in, lift your rib cage, and hold your head high with your chin pointed straight ahead, so you're looking where you are going and not down at your feet. It might feel strange at first, but soon it will start feeling so comfortable you'll wonder how you ever tolerated your slumped posture.

Poor posture can translate into strained, tense muscles in the face. Stand upright, then take a minute to feel where you carry the tension in your body. Most of us carry a lot of tension in our shoulders and necks, so let's start by loosening up those areas.

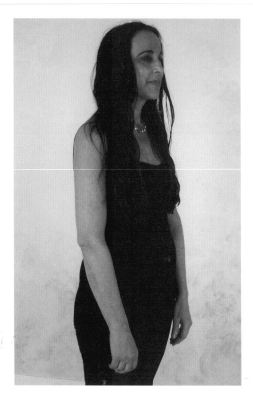

Shoulders Back, Pose 1

Shoulders Back (1)

Stand with feet slightly apart, arms relaxed, and shoulders by the sides of your body. Your arms are probably hanging slightly in front of your body (Pose 1).

Gently rotate the shoulder joint outwards, without lifting your shoulders, so that the palms of your hands face outward (Pose 2). Your spine will straighten naturally, without strain. When it feels comfortable, mentally tell your shoulders this is a better place for them.

Repeat eight times.

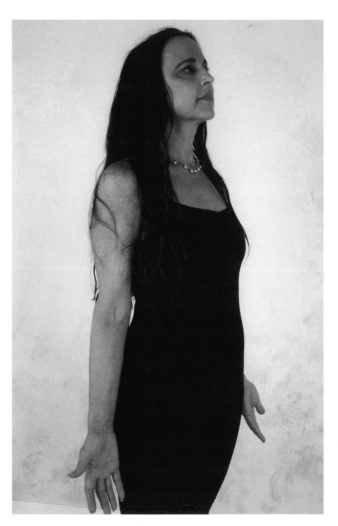

Shoulders Back, Pose 2

Now let's go on to work on some exercises specifically designed to improve circulation, reduce tension, and tone your muscles all at the same time. To develop a healthy complexion your blood circulation must be good. The blood brings nourishment and color into the facial areas and carries away waste matter, helping to prevent acne, blemishes, and wrinkles.

Head and Face—Upside Down (1)

Models sometimes do this simple exercise just before they go before a camera—it's an instant rejuvenator. Besides improving your circulation, the exercise gives you more awareness of your face as part of the whole head. When you think of your face, think of your forehead, scalp, and neck, not just the frontal view. While you are upside down, try to feel where you accumulate tension—some people feel it around the eyes and forehead, others in the jaw and chin area, others in the scalp or neck.

Start standing with your feet about a foot apart, then fold over at the waist. Relax and just let everything drip towards the floor. This position is essentially the same as the first position of the Spine Stretcher/Energizer (Pose 1).

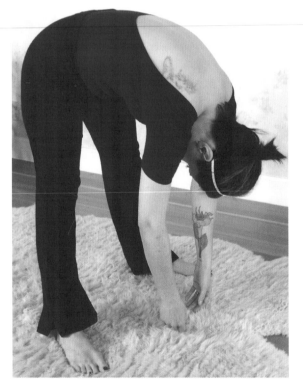

Head and Face—Upside Down, Pose 1

Just so you know, another excellent way to do this exercise is from a sitting position (Pose 2). If you can't leave your chair you can still get the rush!

Another good way to do the upside-down exercise is in front of a full-length mirror. Bend down from the waist and look at your face through your spread legs (Pose 3). Take a few seconds to recover from the shock, then take note of the areas where you will want to work. For example, if your eyes seem to disappear into your cheeks you will want to work on toning sagging cheek areas. You may discover you have multiple chins, so you'll want to include jawline sculpting in your exercise routine. The upside down face is a good way to get started on developing your own exercise routine.

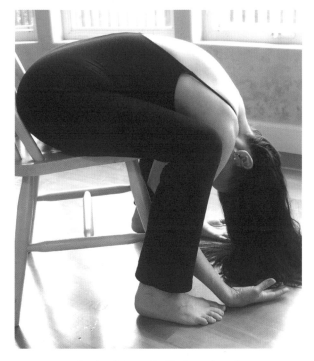

Head and Face—Upside Down, Pose 2

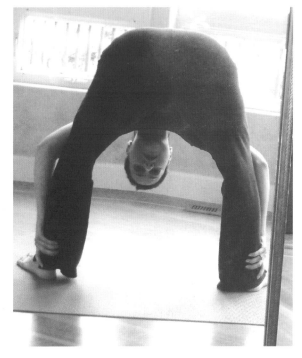

Head and Face—Upside Down, Pose 3

While you're down there, pull gently on your hair, pulling your scalp in a downward direction. Shake your hair—this gets the blood circulating to all areas of your face and scalp. Next comes the good part—return upright and admire how much better you look (Pose 4).

See, it's already working! If you follow your exercise program and do the upside down face at the end of every week you will be rewarded with a brand-new look, even upside down.

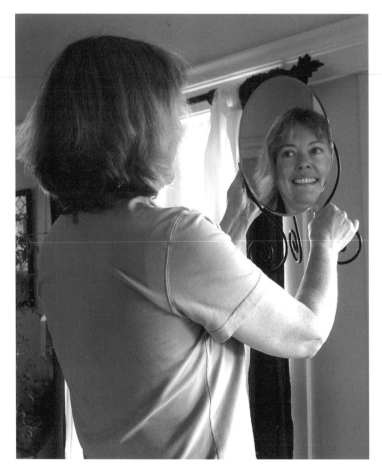

Head and Face—Upside Down, Pose 4

The Lion (1)

The Lion is a well-known yoga pose that exercises all the muscles of your face and neck, even your vocal cords, and is also great for relieving tension. My daughter calls it the "cat coughing up a hair-ball" exercise.

Sit on your heels, resting your hands on your knees.

Now, take a deep breath. On a count of three you are going to do the following all at once: exhale forcefully, make an O with your mouth, then smile without changing the O shape (this forces the cheeks towards the ears), open your eyes wide, and look up (Pose 1).

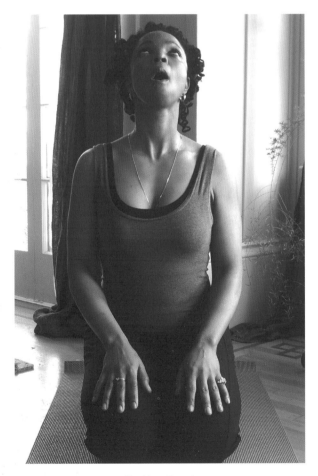

The Lion, Pose 1

Now extend your tongue out and down as far toward your chin as you can, stretch out your fingers, tense them, and say "RRRRRR" as ferociously as you can (Pose 2).

On a count of three, lean forward so your fingertips touch the ground and you're kneeling on your knees. Growl! Growl for a count of ten, then sit back and relax (Pose 3).

Do this two more times.

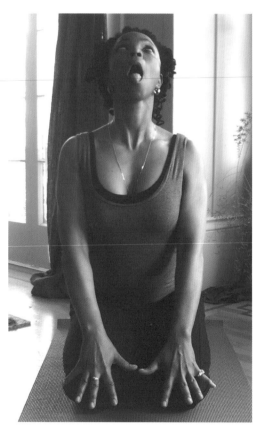

The Lion, Pose 2

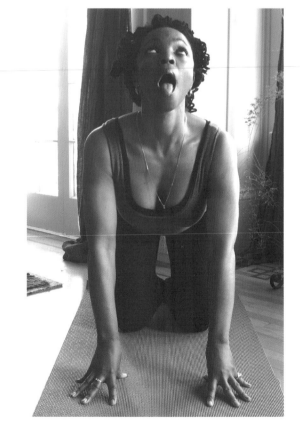

The Lion, Pose 3

Modified Head Stand (2)

This is not nearly as difficult to do as a full-out head stand. If you can do a full head stand, kudos to you—go for it. However, the modified version will also serve to get the blood circulating in the head and neck, so you can be a Yoga Facelift pro even if you can't do the fancy stuff.

Sit on your heels, hold out your arms in front of you, and interlace your fingers, palms facing toward you (Pose 1).

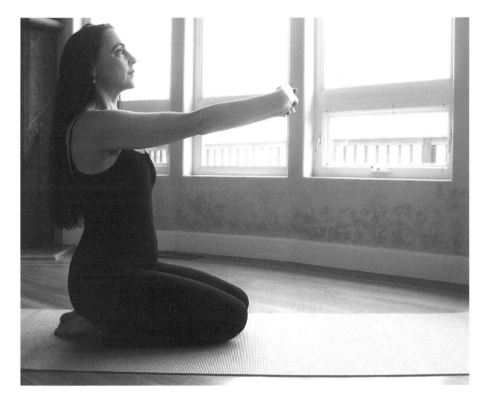

Modified Head Stand, Pose 1

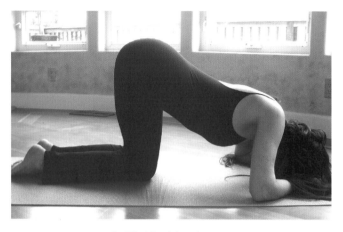

Modified Head Stand, Pose 2

Rise up from your heels, then slowly bend forward and place your elbows and outer edges of your hands on the floor. Your elbows and hands will form a triangle; your elbows are the base corners and your hands are the apex. Lower your head into your clasped hands; allow the front part of your scalp to touch the floor and the back of your head to be cradled by your hands (Pose 2).

Place your full weight on your forearms. Raise your hips, bring knees off the floor, and push up with your toes, so your lower body is off the floor (Pose 3).

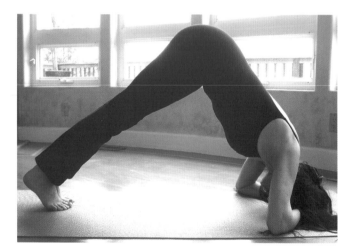

Modified Head Stand, Pose 3

Inch forward slowly with your toes until your knees are as close to your chest as possible (Pose 4). Straighten knees, if possible . Hold this position for a count of thirty. Your weight should be resting primarily on your forearms and hands here—not your head and neck. Be sure to keep the shoulders away from the ears, so the neck stays lengthened (Pose 5).

Lower your knees to the floor, slowly raise your head, rise and bring your hands and arms to your sides and relax into a seated posture.

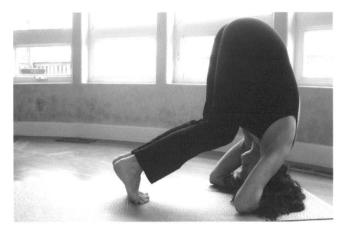

Modified Head Stand, Pose 4

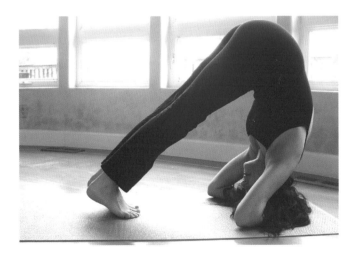

Modified Head Stand, Pose 5

This book includes many neck and chin exercises because these are problem areas for just about everyone. In fact, the neck is the first part of your anatomy to start reflecting your true age.

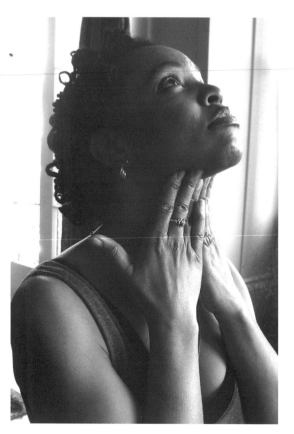

Neck Massage, Pose 1

Neck Massage (1)

This exercise is a great way to tone the neck and firm up that softening jawline. It helps to drain the excess fluid from your neck, prevents sagging, and is a wonderful stress reducer. And it just feels good!

Lift your chin so that your neck forms a taut line. Place your hands together in front of your throat, side by side. Then, with the first three fingers of each hand and starting from your Adam's apple (about two inches below the chin), push the skin of your neck firmly towards the chin (Pose 1).

When you've arrived at your chin, with your right hand push the skin under your jawbone towards your right earlobe, and with the left hand push the skin under the jawbone towards your left earlobe (Pose 2). Use both hands simultaneously, so you are pushing the skin in opposite directions.

Once at the earlobes, massage the neck downward toward the hollows in your collarbone (Pose 3).

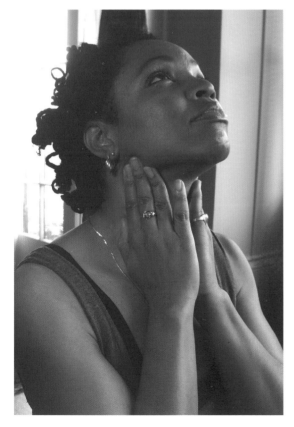

Neck Massage, Pose 2

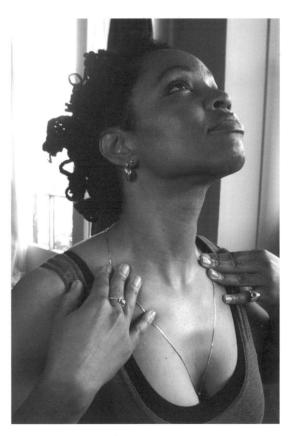

Neck Massage, Pose 3

Chin Lift (1)

You do this one sitting down. It is great for stretching the spine and the neck. This is a wonderful way to get in a good stretch and take a break from your computer without having to leave your office or even your chair.

Sit up straight in your chair. Fold your arms in back so that your forearms are resting along the base of your spine. Push your shoulders down and stretch your neck nice and long (Pose 1).

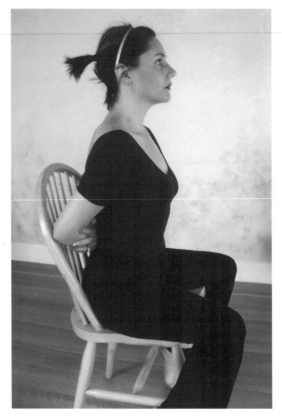

Chin Lift, Pose 1

Now lift your chin up towards the ceiling as high as it will go. Arch your back to really stretch your chin up towards the ceiling, but remember to keep your shoulders down (Pose 2). Look towards the back of the room. Hold the pose for a count of ten.

Slowly release, letting your chin drop to your chest. If you can, stand up for a few seconds to feel what a good stretch this is for your neck and spine.

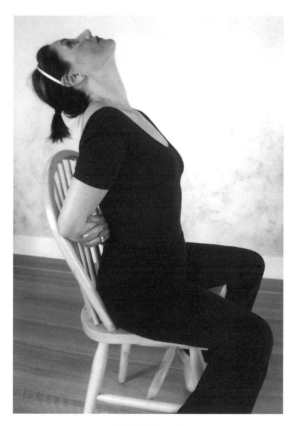

Chin Lift, Pose 2

Head Roll (1)

In a seated posture, close your eyes. Allow your head to come forward and rest your chin against your chest (Pose 1). Hold for a count of ten.

Very slowly roll your head to the extreme left position and hold without motion for a count of ten (Pose 2).

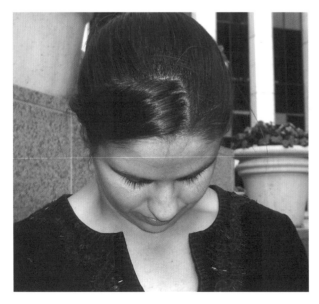

Head Roll, Pose 1

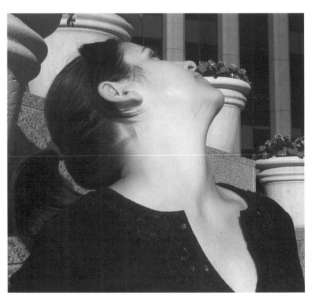

Head Roll, Pose 2

Very slowly roll your head to the extreme backward position and hold for a count of ten (Pose 3).

Very slowly roll your head to the extreme right position and hold for a count of ten (Pose 4).

Very slowly roll your head to the front position so that your head rests against your chest again for a count of ten (Pose 1). Repeat the movements, but this time clockwise, starting with the extreme right position. Repeat twice.

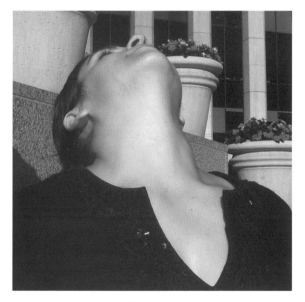

Head Roll, Pose 3

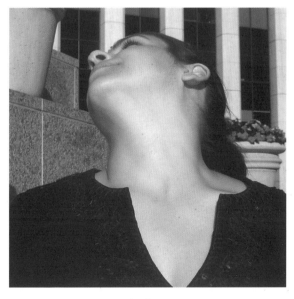

Head Roll, Pose 4

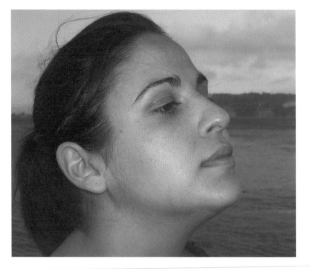

Neck I, Pose 1

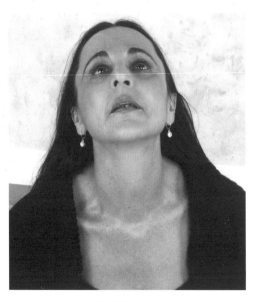

Neck II, Pose 1

Neck I (1)

Lift your chin to create a taut line.

Press the top of your tongue against the roof of your mouth. Your mouth may fall open slightly. Hold for ten seconds (Pose 1).

Repeat three times, holding each time for a count of ten.

Neck II (1)

Lift your chin to create a taut line.

Press your back teeth together while you press the tip of your tongue against the inside of your lower gum line (Pose 1). Your mouth may be slightly open. Hold for ten seconds. Rest.

Repeat three times, holding each time for a count of ten.

Head Twist (2)

You can do this one sitting or standing up.

Clasp your hands and rest them firmly on the back of your head. Gently push down with your clasped hands until your chin is pressing firmly against your chest (Pose 1). Hold for a count of ten.

Slowly raise your head and rest your chin in your left palm. Place your right hand firmly on the back of your head. Use your hands to turn your head slowly as far to the left as possible (Pose 2). Hold for a count of five.

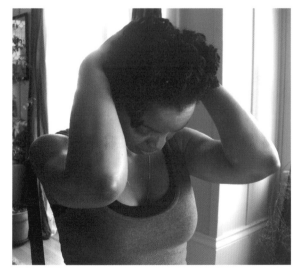

Head Twist, Pose 1

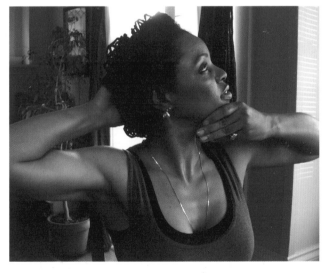

Head Twist, Pose 2

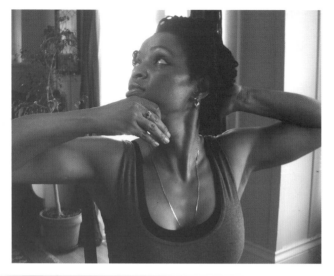

Head Twist, Pose 3

Remove your hands, but keep your head in the same position. Then use your hands to push your head left as far as possible once again.

Hold for a count of five, then release, but keep your head in place. Then use your hands to push your head to the left one last time. Release and relax, allowing your head to return to center and drop towards your chest.

Your head should twist a little farther back each time, but remember, *never* push your head so far that it causes discomfort. Always be very gentle when doing neck exercises.

Now turn your head with your hands as far to the right as possible (Pose 3).

Hold for a count of five. Remove hands briefly, then once again use your hands to push your head right as far as possible. Hold again for a count of five. Release and repeat once more. Rest your chin on your chest and relax.

Repeat the entire exercise—to the center, to the left, and to the right—one more time.

Keep Your Chin Up (2)

This exercise is very similar to the Head Roll, but with an added twist that puts it in the intermediate category. If you have any jaw or TMJ (temporomandibular joint) problems, do not do this exercise —just stay with the simple head roll.

In a comfortable seated or standing posture allow your jaw to slacken and go completely limp, so your mouth is open. Protrude your jaw and raise it very slowly until your bottom teeth are over the upper front teeth (Pose 1).

As in the Head Roll, turn your head to the right and look up (Pose 2). Hold for a count of ten. Then tilt your head all the way back while still protruding your jaw, and hold for a count of ten. Then turn your head to the left, keeping your jaw protruded, and hold for a count of ten. Return your head to the starting position, then relax and slowly lower your jaw. Do the same thing again in a counterclockwise direction.

Repeat the entire sequence one more time.

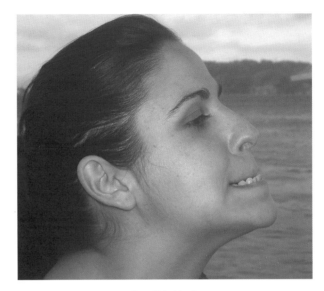

Keep Your Chin Up, Pose 1

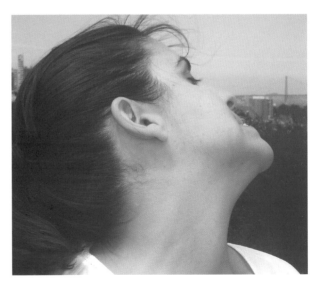

Keep Your Chin Up, Pose 2

Cow Face for the Neck and Chin (3)

Allow your jaw to slacken and go completely limp so your mouth is open. Protrude your jaw and raise it very slowly until your bottom teeth are over your upper front teeth (Pose 1).

Get into Cow Face position, starting with the right arm raised.

Turn your head to the left and look up (Pose 2). Hold for a count of five. Slowly lower and relax your jaw, but keep your arms in place. Lift and protrude your jaw again, this time holding for a count of ten.

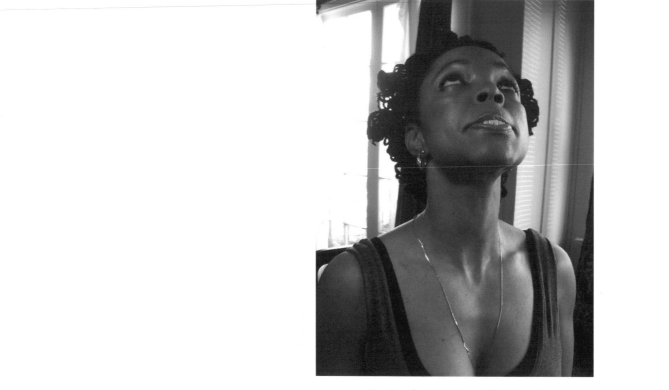

Cow Face for the Neck and Chin, Pose 1

Repeat two more times on the left side. The last time, release your jaw, lower your head and arms, and relax. Take a deep breath. Then repeat the same sequence on the left side.

Now we'll do the same exercise for the other side. This time, raise your left arm and reach toward the back with your left hand while you reach around with your right hand. Protrude your jaw, then repeat the series of head movements, turning to the right this time.

After the third time, relax your arms and take a deep breath.

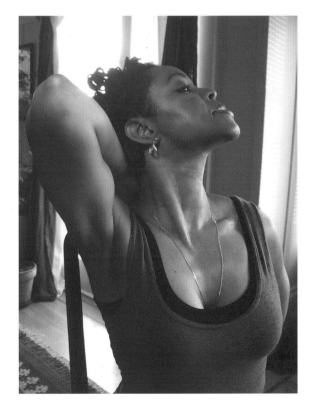

Cow Face for the Neck and Chin, Pose 2

Neck Stretch and Back Bend (3)

You may do this exercise standing or kneeling. It firms the neck and lifts the forehead and eyebrows.

Kneel on the floor or stand erect. Bend your head forward so it rests on your chest (Pose 1). Hold for a count of ten.

Slowly lift your head upright then backward until you are looking at the wall in back of you. Now arch your spine backward as far as you comfortably can, as if you are trying to see the floor in back of you. Keep your hips and thighs forward as much as possible. Put your hands on the small of your back or on the backs of your thighs for support (Pose 2). Keep your eyes open. Your neck is stretched and taut. Hold for a count of ten. Return to your original position and take a deep breath.

Repeat twice more.

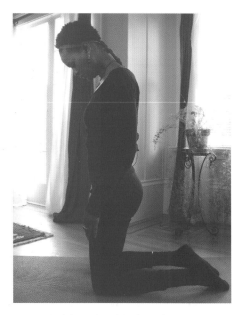

Neck Stretch and Back Bend, Pose 1

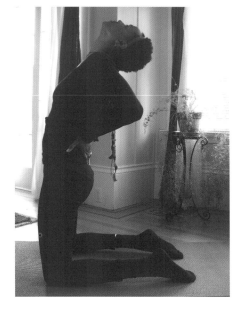

Neck Stretch and Back Bend, Pose 2

The Jawline

As we get older our jawline starts to lose its definition, and we may even develop jowls or dewlaps. These exercises will do wonders to firm up that whole area, taking years off the face.

Jawline Definer (1)

Place your index fingers on the inside of your mouth, resting alongside your bottom molars, toward the back where the jaw hinges (Pose 1). Clench your teeth together and push your jaw muscles in against the resistance of your fingers. Hold for a count of five, then release. These are the muscles you chew with, and you can feel how powerful they are as you work them.

Repeat five times.

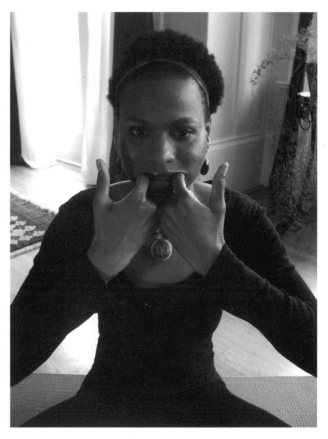

Jawline Definer, Pose 1

Jawline Sculptor (1)

Starting from the tips of the earlobes, lightly grasp the flesh on both sides of your jawline between your fingertips, using small pinching movements, working towards the chin (Poses 1, 2). As you pinch lightly, tighten the muscles of the neck. Feel the resistance against your fingers.

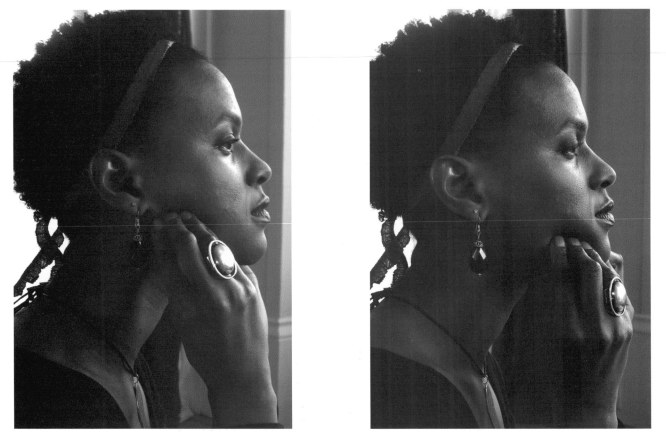

Jawline Sculptor, Pose 1

Jawline Sculptor, Pose 2

When you get to the chin area, hold your thumbs right under the tip of your chin. Push the muscle at the tip of your chin down against your thumbs, feeling the muscle of your chin tighten as you do (Pose 3). This is your platysmus, and if it is not exercised you may end up with a loose fold of skin under your chin, often referred to as the "turkey wattle." Push ten times, then relax. Starting from the chin, repeat the pinching movements back towards the earlobes.

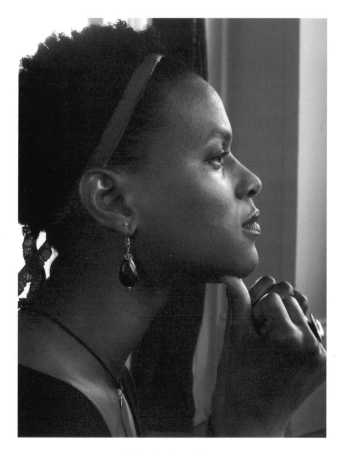

Jawline Sculptor, Pose 3

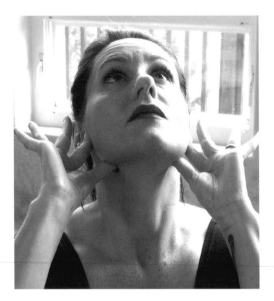

Jawline Massage, Pose 1

Jawline Massage (1)

In the Jawline Sculptor you pinch the flesh between your fingers. This exercise is only slightly different—here you massage the neck and under-jaw area rather than pinching the flesh. In both exercises you really work the masseter and temporalis muscles (see diagram on page 21) against the resistance of your fingers.

Starting from your earlobes, use your thumbs and index fingers and feel for your jawline (Pose 1).

Work your way toward your chin, using the fingers of each hand (Pose 2). This is an isometric exercise, and in this case you are contracting the muscles of your chin and neck. You are using your fingers to help feel your muscles working. Push your chin downward as you gently push upward with your fingers, and push your neck outward as you push your fingers gently inward. You do not need to apply strong pressure with your fingers. Just use them to feel the muscles contracting.

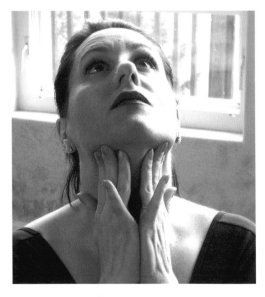

Jawline Massage, Pose 2

When you reach your chin, feel for your platysmus muscle, that little muscle right under your chin that gives you that turkey wattle. Curl your fingers of one hand to make a half fist and place your first two curled fingers under your chin right on the muscle (Pose 3). Push down with your chin against your fist. Push for a fast count of ten, then relax.

Repeat the whole sequence of pushing against the jaw again, starting from your chin and moving back towards your ears.

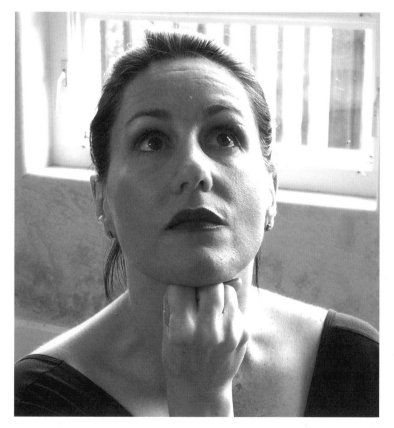

Jawline Massage, Pose 3

Jawline Shaper (1)

Curl your fingers to make a half fist with each hand. Place both half fists under your chin so that the little fingers of each hand meet in the middle of your neck, alongside the underside of your jaw (Pose 1).

Push your chin down against your fists.

Contract and relax the chin and neck muscles, so that your chin is pushing down against your fists, for a count of ten. Feel those neck muscles work. Then relax. Contract and relax your muscles for a quick count of ten, then relax.

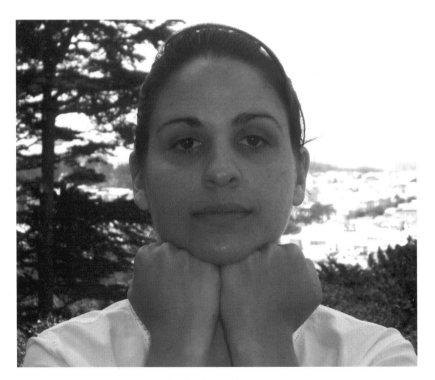

Jawline Shaper, Pose 1

Now move your two hands slightly apart (Pose 2). Contract and release the neck muscles again for another count of ten.

Now move your hands slightly apart once more—the curled fingers are resting on the sides of your neck, under the jawline. Contract and release the muscles for a final count of ten. Relax.

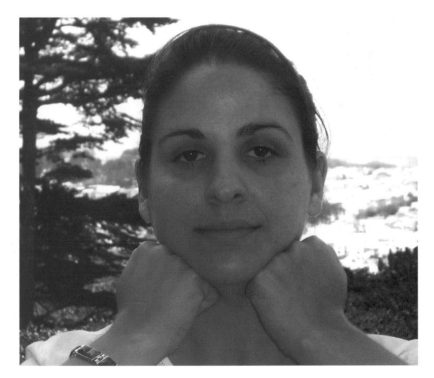

Jawline Shaper, Pose 2

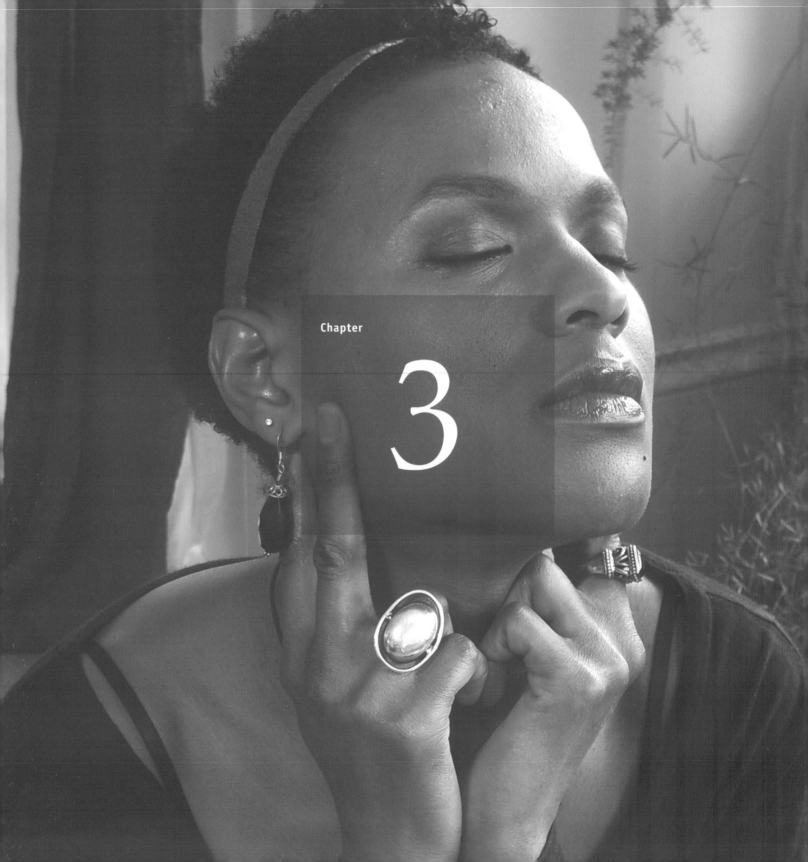

Chapter

3

Exercises for Specific Areas

Cheekbone Creator (1)

This exercise targets saggy cheeks and, incidentally, helps to reveal beautiful cheekbones in people who didn't know they had any. According to a friend of mine this exercise also helps open up her nasal passages, and she is able to breathe more easily. It is also wonderful to do if you have sinus problems. Just do this simple exercise whenever you want instant relief.

Put your anchor fingers (your two forefingers) of each hand just outside your nostrils (Pose 1). Smile without smiling, drawing your cheeks up. Open your eyes wide. Hold for count of ten.

Release.

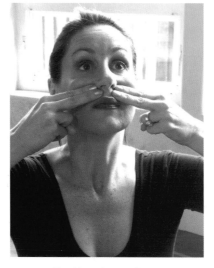

Cheekbone Creator, Pose 1

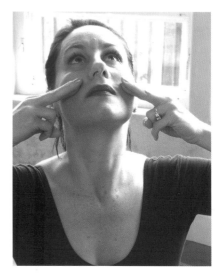

Cheekbone Creator, Pose 2

Move your fingers outward until they rest on the middle of your cheeks. Push up gently until you feel your cheekbones (Pose 2). Open your eyes wide, smile without smiling, hold for a count of ten.

Move your fingers farther apart so that now they rest on the hollow between your cheekbone and your jaw (Pose 3). Holding your mouth slightly open, press in and up with your fingers, toward your ears, holding for a count of ten. Keep your jaws separated and don't clench your teeth.

For Droopy Cheeks (2)

Place your index finger just in front of your right ear, on your temple, between the edge or your right eyebrow and your hairline. Curl your finger slightly (Pose 1). Move your cheek up and back toward your fingers, making the line along your nasal-labial fold (sometimes called the "marionette" line—the fine crease that curves around one side of your mouth) disappear. Do this ten times in quick succession.

Relax. Go to the other side and do the same thing.

Relax, then repeat one more time for each side.

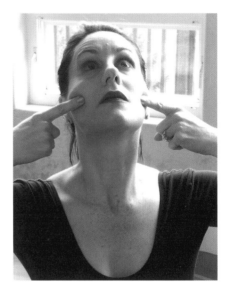

Cheekbone Creator, Pose 3

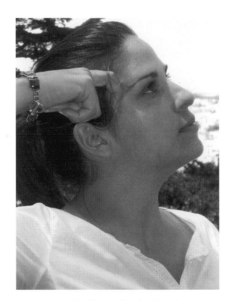

For Droopy Cheeks, Pose 1

Erasing Marionette Lines (3)

This exercise is good for softening those nasal-labial fold lines (the marionette lines).

Crook your left forefinger and place it along the right nasal-labial fold. The left thumb goes in the mouth. Pinch thumb and forefinger together to anchor the muscles. Place the forefinger of your right hand on your temple in front of your right ear (Pose 1).

Contract your right cheek muscles up and towards your ear. With a pulsing movement that can be felt around your temples, pull your cheek muscles up towards the ear for a count of ten. Relax, then repeat twice more.

Repeat the same movements for the same count on the right side.

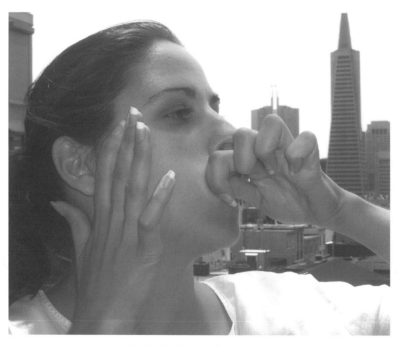

Erasing Marionette Lines, Pose 1

Lips and Mouth

Upper Lip Line Eraser (1)

This exercise addresses those pesky lines along the upper lip. It works best as a preventive measure, but it will also help with existing lines.

Place the inside tip of one forefinger just above your top lip and the inside tip of the other forefinger just underneath your bottom lip (Pose 1) to feel the tingle in your orbicularis oris (the muscle surrounding the mouth area). Keep lips relaxed while stimulating the muscle and feeling the energy.

Switch fingers and do the same thing (Pose 2).

Repeat two times.

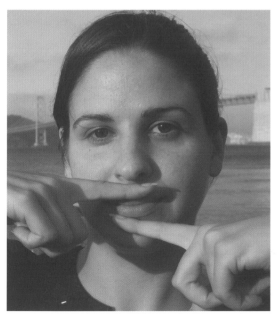

Upper Lip Line Eraser, Pose 1

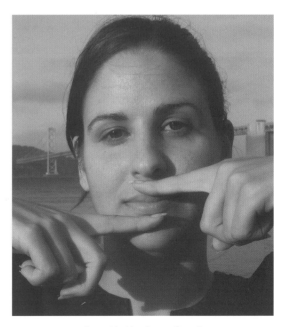

Upper Lip Line Eraser, Pose 2

Upper Lip Smoothie (1)

This exercise strengthens the top part of your orbicularis oris. If you have a tendency to pucker your lips, which creates so-called "smoker's lines" around them, use this exercise to help you visualize a smooth upper lip that you wouldn't dream of puckering.

Place your forefingers on either side of your mouth corners to anchor the muscles. Stretch your top lip down and over your top teeth and toward your mouth corners at the same time (Pose 1). Your upper lip should be completely smooth, no puckers. Hold for a count of five, then release. Repeat three times, holding for a count of ten each time.

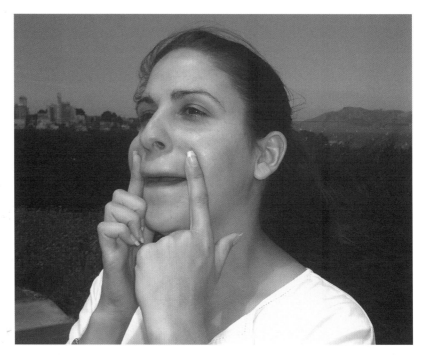

Upper Lip Smoothie, Pose 1

The Carp Curl (2)

The philtrum (the area between the nose and the top lip) starts to lengthen and the top lip starts to disappear as we get older. This carp curl exercise counteracts that tendency.

Place your two forefingers on either side above your mouth, along the nasal-labial folds. This serves to stabilize the area as you work your orbicularis oris. Without making lines in your upper lip—stretch it forward—curl it up towards your nose, as if you were lifting a weight with it (Pose 1). Curl your lip up and out, as if you are a fish sucking in water. Curl it ten times, relax, then curl it ten times more, this time a bit faster. Curl it another ten times, this time faster still. Relax.

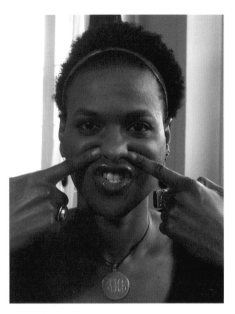

The Carp Curl, Pose 1

The Carp Curl—Advanced (3)

Place your forefingers on either side above your mouth, along the nasal-labial folds, and curl your lip toward your nose as in the previous exercise.

Now stretch your upper lip down over your teeth (Pose 1). Repeat the two movements so that you resemble a fish. Repeat ten times. Relax.

Now do it ten times again, only a little faster. Relax.

Now do it once more, just a little faster. Feel the burn. You may also feel the contraction in your cheeks, which is fine.

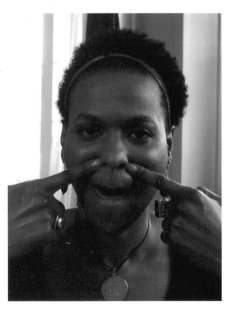

The Carp Curl—Advanced, Pose 1

Palming (1)

This exercise is a must for people who work long hours in front of the computer. It is great for reducing puffiness around the eyes, and is very soothing for the optic nerve as well as the eye in general.

Find a comfortable seated position, either on the floor on a cushion or in a chair. Sit with your back straight. Begin with your eyes closed. Focus on your breath as it moves in and out of your nostrils. Cool air in, warm air out.

Now rub your palms together very fast until they feel warm (Pose 1). Then cup them over your closed eyes, so that the heels of your hands are directly over the eyeballs (Pose 2). Contract your orbicularis oculi (the muscle that surrounds your eyes) against the heel of your hand. Feel it pushing against your hand.

Contract and release ten times. Rest. Repeat five times.

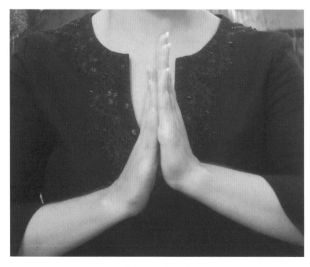

Palming, Pose 1

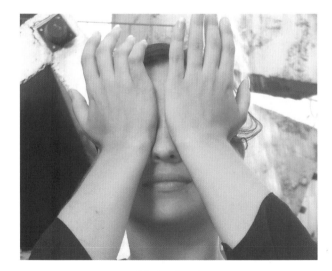

Palming, Pose 2

Lower Eye (1)

This exercise tones the muscle around the eye, the orbicularis oculi, and consequently helps to smooth out crow's feet.

Make V's with the first two fingers of both hands. Place the fingertips of the forefingers on the outer corner of each eye. The second fingers rest on each side of the inner corner of each eye (Pose 1).

Raise and lower the bottom lids rapidly (Pose 2). This is almost like a blink, but try to keep your eyes open, if you can. "Blink" ten times. Stop, then repeat two more times.

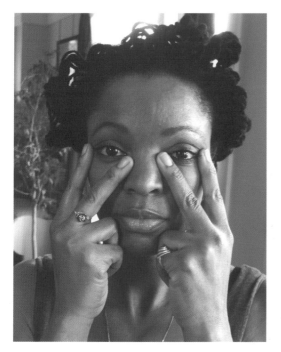

Lower Eye, Pose 1

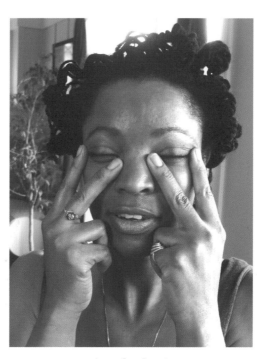

Lower Eye, Pose 2

Upper Eye (2)

This exercise targets the upper part of the eye, under the eyebrow. It does wonders to prevent eyelid wrinkles and forestall the "crepeiness" that starts to appear in this area.

Place the four fingertips of each hand on each eyebrow, pushing eyebrows up very slightly (Pose 1). Close your eyes, then tighten your upper lids while pushing them against your fingertips. Hold for a count of ten.

Repeat twice.

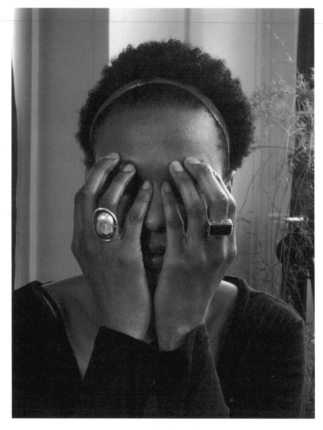

Upper Eye, Pose 1

For Crow's Feet and Puffy Eyes (2)

Practice this very relaxing eye soother at the end of a workday or whenever you need a break.

Make sideways V's with forefinger and middle finger of each hand. Place your forefingers on your top lids, pushing up the brows slightly. Place your middle fingers on the bottom lids (Pose 1).

Contract your orbicularis oculi muscle against your fingertips. Hold for one to two seconds. Release.

Now close the V until your two fingers are together over the center of your eye. Your forefingers are resting against your top lids, the middle fingers are resting on your bottom lids (Pose 2).

Again, contract your orbicularis oculi muscle against your fingertips. Hold for one to two seconds. Release.

Press gently against your eyeballs for a few seconds and release, then open your eyes slowly and blink.

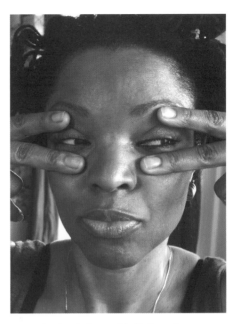

For Crow's Feet and Puffy Eyes, Pose 1

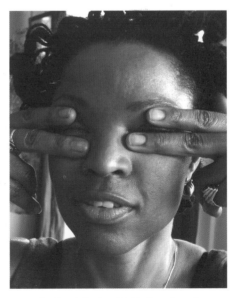

For Crow's Feet and Puffy Eyes, Pose 2

For Upper Eyelids (2)

As we get older the space between the brow and the top of the eye tends to shorten. This is another exercise to help strengthen the muscle under the eyebrow, which helps to prevent sagging in that area.

Curve both of your forefingers into upside down L's. Place them along your upper eye bone, just under your eyebrow (Pose 1).

Press fingers gently against the bone. Contract the muscles of your upper eyelids against your fingers. Do this ten times.

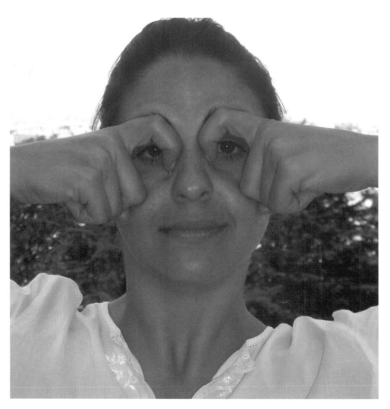

For Upper Eyelids, Pose 1

Eye Socket Massage and Crow's Feet Extinguisher (3)

Take your index or middle finger of each hand and place them on either side of your nose just below the bridge (Pose 1). Move your fingers up the bridge of your nose and along the bone underneath your eyebrows. You'll feel a notch under your brows where the bone begins to turn downward. Rub the notch gently for a moment (Pose 2).

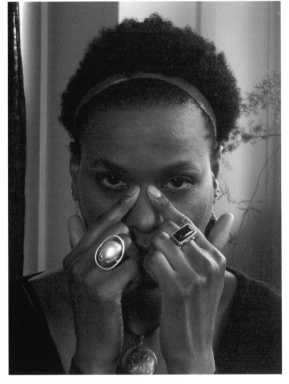

Eye Socket Massage and Crow's Feet Extinguisher, Pose 1

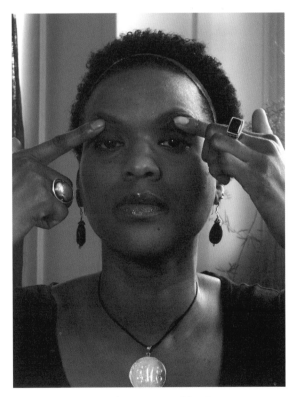

Eye Socket Massage and Crow's Feet Extinguisher, Pose 2

Now follow the eye bone to the outer corner of your left eye. Take your left index finger and place it against the outer corner of your left eye, making sure you are flattening the lines. Make a sideways V with the first two fingers of your right hand. Place the right forefinger underneath your left eyebrow and the right middle finger underneath the middle of eye, anchoring the muscles (Pose 3). Contract your lower lid against the resistance of all three fingers (Pose 4). This is almost like a blink, but keep your eyes open. You should be moving only the lower lid.

Repeat eight times for each eye.

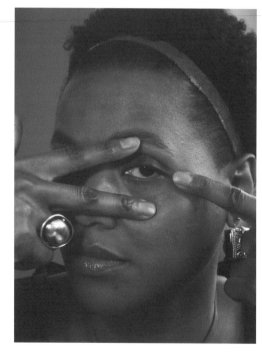

Eye Socket Massage and Crow's Feet
Extinguisher, Pose 3

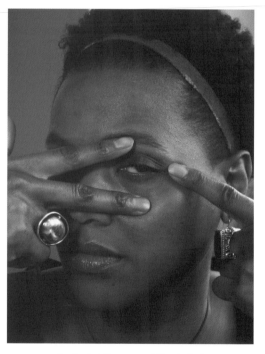

Eye Socket Massage and Crow's Feet
Extinguisher, Pose 4

For Droopy Eyes (3)

This exercise takes some concentration, but it is extremely effective for giving a lift to the eyes at the corners.

Place forefingers of each hand on either side of the outer corners of each eye, so that the sides of the fingers rest against the forehead just in front of the hairline (Pose 1). Without making lines in your forehead, move the muscles surrounding your eyes up towards your fingertips. Hold for a count of five, then release.

Repeat five times.

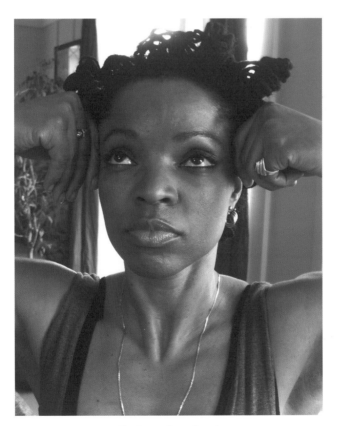

For Droopy Eyes, Pose 1

Tension Banisher (1)

Many of my students have told me that this exercise is the one to do if you have a tension headache.

Place the index and middle fingers of both hands in the middle of your forehead. Rub your forehead by making feathering motions with your fingers (Pose 1).

Now raise your scalp and forehead by lifting your brows slightly with your fingertips. Hold that position while you massage your forehead in short, upward strokes towards your hairline (Pose 2). Release. Alternate feathering and stroking six times.

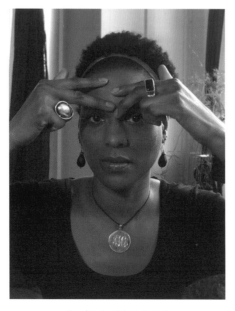

Tension Banisher, Pose 1

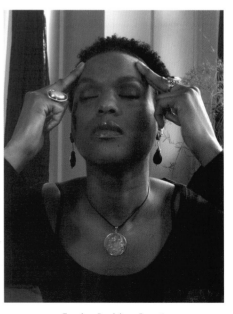

Tension Banisher, Pose 2

Move your fingers across your brow to your temples, pausing there to give your temples a gentle massage. This is an area where we hold stress and tension that can often lead to headaches.

Then move your fingers to the corners of your eyes and massage gently (Pose 3).

Move your fingers down to the hinge of your jaw, pausing to massage your jaw muscles (Pose 4). Then move your fingers along your jawline, massaging firmly.

Move your fingers down to your collarbone. Then, turning your head to the right, massage both sides of your neck with firm upward strokes (Pose 5). Turn your head to the left and repeat the massage on the left side of your neck.

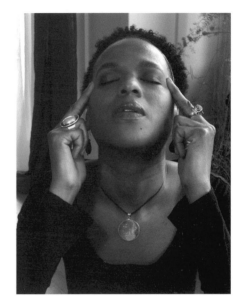

Tension Banisher, Pose 3

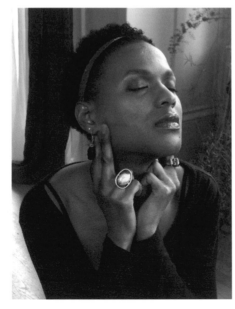

Tension Banisher, Pose 4

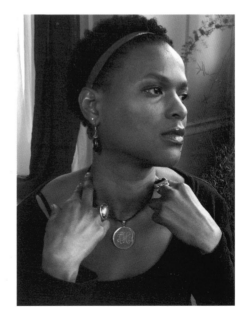

Tension Banisher, Pose 5

Scalp Tingler (1)

With both hands on the top of your head, reach deeply into the roots of your hair and firmly grasp as much hair as you can hold. Pull up, making your scalp wiggle (Pose 1). Do this ten times. Do not make wrinkles in your forehead while you are doing this.

Now move your hands to the sides of your head and pull hair upwards and backwards for a count of ten (Pose 2). I call this the "facelift pull," because this is the area plastic surgery addresses when a facelift is done. Of course, you're much better off toning those muscles all on your own.

Now move your hands to the back of your scalp and pull hair backwards for a count of ten (Pose 3).

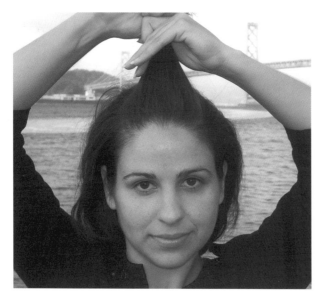

Scalp Tingler, Pose 1

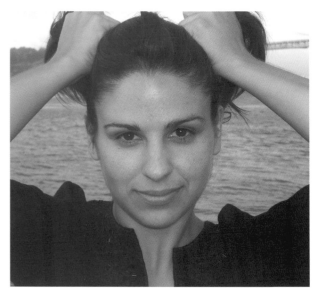

Scalp Tingler, Pose 2

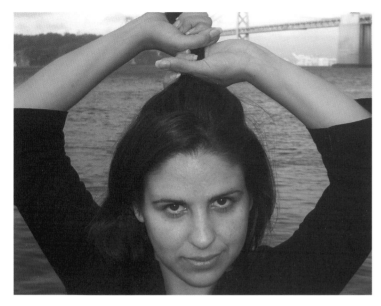

Scalp Tingler, Pose 3

Counteracting Vertical Lines (the Scowl Lines)

The scowl lines appear between your brows as one or two deep furrows. They are sometimes called the Botox lines because these are the lines most commonly addressed with Botox injections. You realize just how powerful these muscles, called the corrugator muscles, are when you see yourself or others with deep lines in this area. Scowling or squinting too much creates these lines, and you can see them even on young people who've acquired this bad habit. Here are some tips to help prevent them, or, if you already have them, to help soften them.

1. A common cause of scowling is simply squinting because you can't see properly. If you find yourself doing that, it's time to have your eyes checked.

2. We make about 50 percent of our expression lines, and the scowl lines in particular, when we are sleeping. We don't realize when we're dreaming how often we scowl, frown, or make other faces. Putting Scotch tape over the scowl lines before we go to bed actually reminds us not to make those expressions while we're sleeping.

3. Use the Scowl Banisher exercise (see page 82) to train the corrugators to pull apart the brows rather than pull them together.

Counteracting Horizontal Lines (2)

Place the four fingertips of each hand along the upper hairline and push up gently (Pose 1). Pull your forehead muscles down towards your eyes against the resistance of your fingertips. Hold for a count of ten.

Repeat two more times.

Scowl Banisher (2)

This is an exercise that requires some concentration—just don't scowl or frown while you're concentrating!

Feel the movement of pulling your eyebrows together (Pose 1). Painful, isn't it?

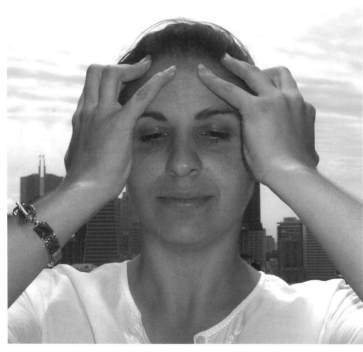

Counteracting Horizontal Lines, Pose 1

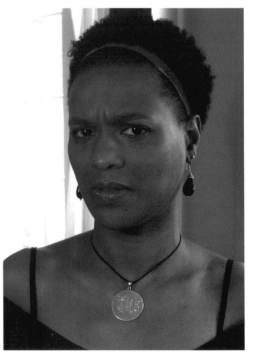

Scowl Banisher, Pose 1

Now place your fingertips on either side of the scowl line. Pull your fingers gently apart to smooth out the line. Now try to pull your brows together, but be careful to avoid making the line again (Pose 2). You are strengthening the muscles around the line, not deepening the line itself. Hold for a count of ten.

Now move your fingers further apart so that they rest in the middle of your forehead, approximately above the arch of each eyebrow. Contract your forehead muscles outward toward your fingers and your temples, pulling that vertical line smooth (Pose 3).

Alternate Poses 2 and 3 one more time.

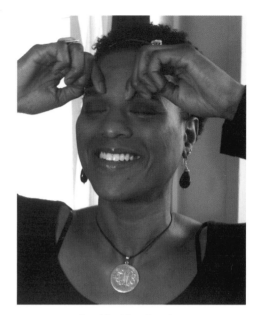

Scowl Banisher, Pose 2

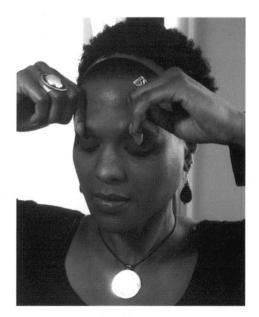

Scowl Banisher, Pose 3

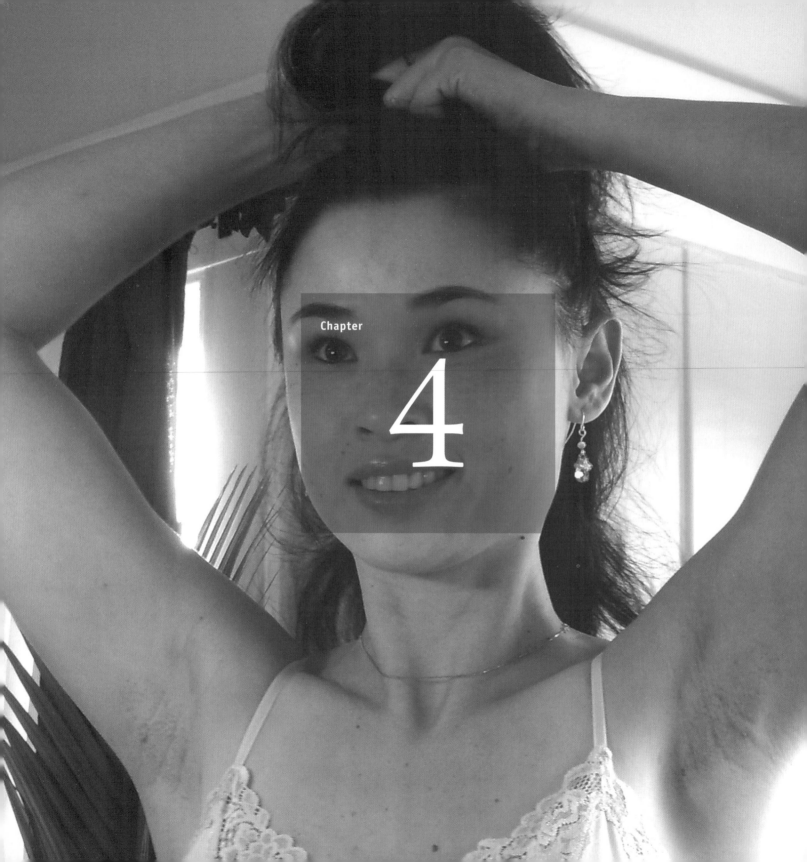

Chapter

4

The Facelift Series

This is my favorite series of intermediate exercises. The exercises combine physical movement with mental focus, and are very effective at creating lift in the entire face. I've placed all the exercises in chapter four in the intermediate category for a reason. When you first start doing the Yoga Facelift, you are working to acquire awareness of the muscles of the face, and practicing exercises that will help you learn to control some of those 190 facial muscles. Once you've had a little practice, you will be ready to build on that knowledge.

Muscle Memory

We've all had the experience of being able to find a location we've been to just by making the physical movments we took before to get there. For example, when we walk to our neighborhood grocery store (or the park, or even just around the block if you are just beginning to wean yourself away from automobile tyranny) we don't have to think, "Now I make a right here, and then go two blocks and make a left at the witch's house"; we don't have to *think* about it at all, our bodies just take over. This is because all muscles have memory—even facial muscles. The beginner's job is to create a new set of memories for facial muscles to draw upon. You will be amazed at how quickly you can accomplish this—new habits replace old ones very rapidly. After a few exercise sessions, you will find that your muscles have incorporated the new memories, and you will have acquired a whole new set of facial habits. When you have done this, you will be ready to build on your new skills with the exercises in chapter four, where the focus shifts from doing purely mechanical exercises to energetics and visualization.

Facelift I (2)

Step One: Stand comfortably, looking straight ahead. Now concentrate on tightening your cheek muscles—do this by making an O with your mouth, then, without changing the shape of your mouth, move your cheek muscles up and back towards your ears as you would if you were smiling. You may place your forefingers on each side of your mouth to anchor your lips (Pose I). Hold for a count of five. Release.

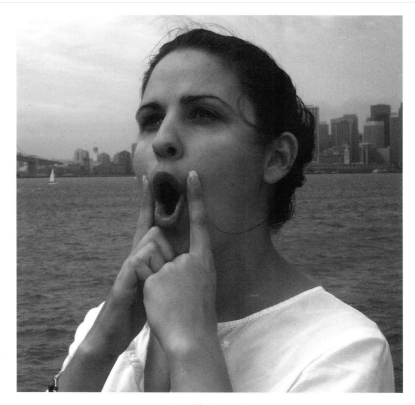

Facelift I, Pose 1

Step Two: Bend over at the waist. Shake your cheeks gently. Now tighten your cheeks the same way you did in the previous step, while you were standing up. Hold for a count of twenty.

Without releasing your cheek muscles, come slowly back up to a standing position. This takes some concentration. Now release. Take a deep breath.

Do Step Two twice more. Remember, gravity is your friend when you are upside down, but it's not really your pal when you are upright.

Facelift II (2)

This one works to lift eyes and forehead. As we get older the distance between our eyebrows and our eyes shortens—we're going to work on widening the gap.

Step One: Stand comfortably, looking straight ahead. Relax your face. With your fingers, just feel the placement of your eyebrows. Take hold of a large portion of hair on the top of your head and pull gently upwards (Pose 1). Visualize what is happening to the upper part of your face—your eyes are wider, your brows are lifted, your fore-head is smooth.

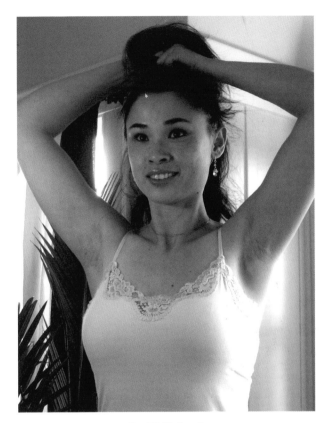

Facelift II, Pose 1

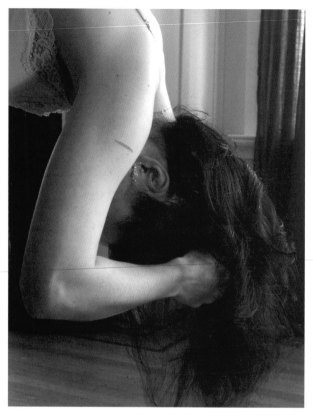

Facelift II, Pose 2

Let go of your hair. Now we're going to do the same thing upside down.

Step Two: Bend over at the waist. Feel how gravity pulls your whole face upward. Feel the placement of your eyebrows. Grasp your hair again and tug, focusing on keeping all the muscles in your forehead and scalp taut (Pose 2). Hold for a count of twenty.

Without releasing your muscles and with your hands still in your hair, come slowly back up to a standing position. When you release, visualize your eyebrows staying in their new position.

Do Step Two twice more.

Facelift III (2)

Step One: Stand comfortably, looking straight ahead. Relax your face. Starting at your collarbone, bring your hands up along the sides of your face, but without actually touching your face (Pose 1). Visualize everything moving up—feel it in your cheeks, forehead, and scalp.

Bring your fingertips together about five inches above your head. Imagine that you have strings leading from your fingers to the top of your head. You've created an energy field around your face, and all the muscles are stretching in the direction of your fingers. Remember that image. Bring your hands down.

Step Two: Bend over at the waist. Starting with your hands at your collarbone, make that the same energy field with your hands. With your hands hovering above the top of your head (your fingertips do not need to be touching), feel all your muscles being pulled by the invisible strings leading from your hands. Feel how gravity pulls your whole face upward. Hold for a count of twenty.

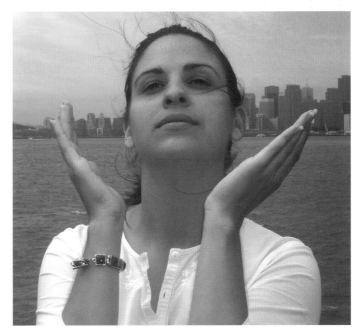

Facelift III, Pose 1

Keeping your hands in the same position, come slowly back up to standing (Pose 2). You should feel your whole scalp tingle. Bring your hands back to your side. Take a deep breath.

Do this step twice more. Now that you've created a lovely force field that looks like a shimmery bubble all around your head and neck, try to maintain awareness of it throughout the rest of your exercise routine.

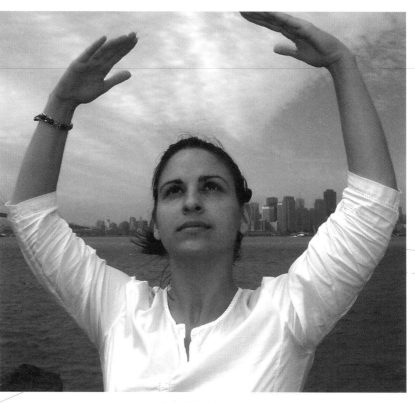

Facelift III, Pose 2

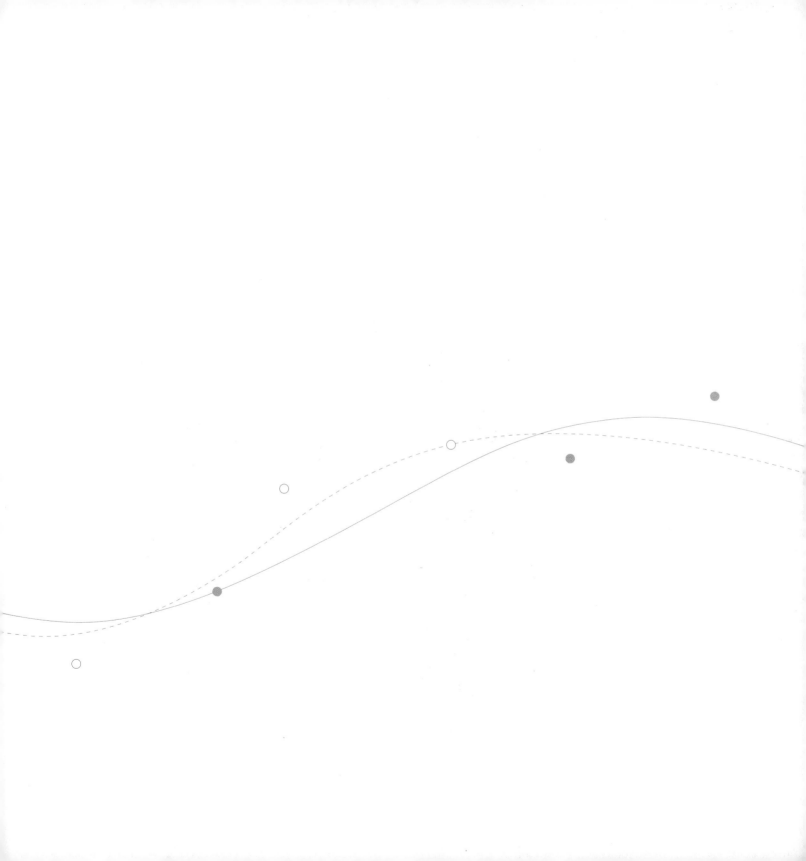

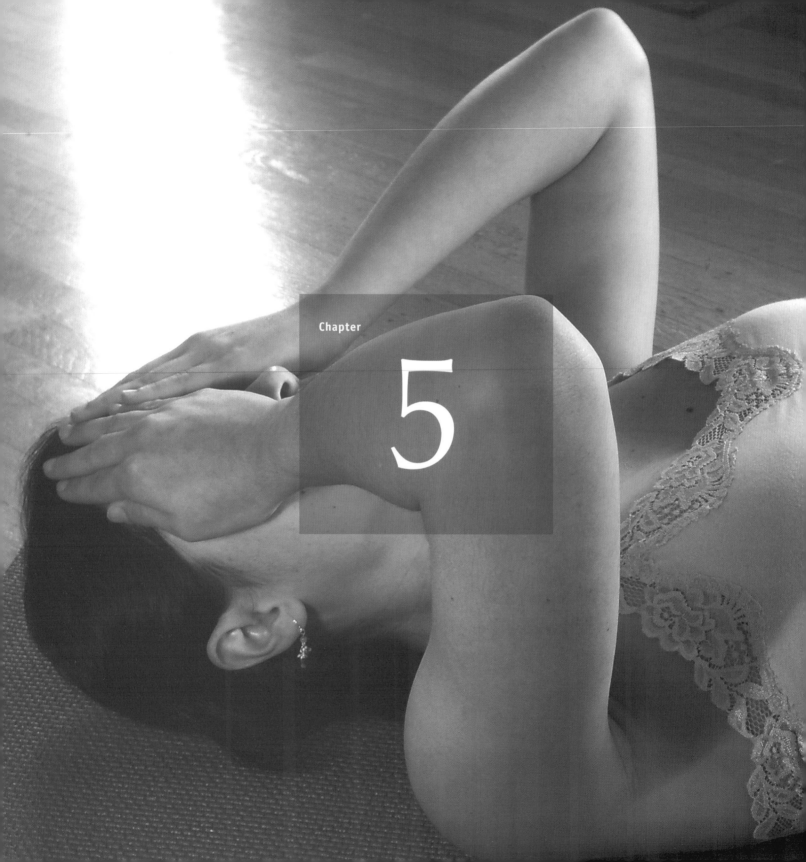

Chapter

5

Relaxation and Rejuvenation

It's a good idea to end an exercise routine with a cool down. It will help you prepare for the day, or if you are preparing for sleep, it is an excellent way to usher in pleasant dreams.

Relaxation (1)

Lie down and relax. If you can't lie down but you still want to take a ten-minute relaxation break, you can also do this exercise sitting.

First, focus on your breath as it moves in and out of your nostrils. Cool air in, warm air out. Breathe deeply and rhythmically.

Now rub your palms together very fast until they feel warm. Then cup them over your closed eyes (Pose 1). This pose is great for puffy eyes and very soothing for both the optic nerve and the eyes in general.

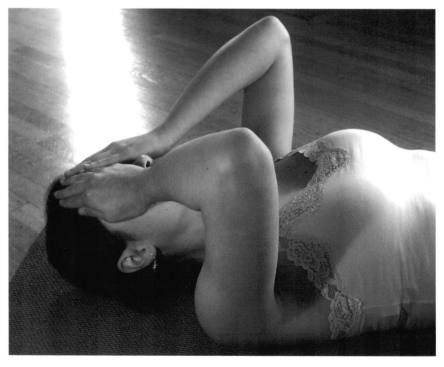

Relaxation, Pose 1

With your hands over your eyes, visualize a rainbow-colored force field around your head and neck. All the muscles of your face feel tingly and alive. Recall the exercises you did that gave you the facial expressions you wanted to convey to the world. Breathe deeply and enjoy the sensation of peace, rest, and quiet. Remove your hands and relax completely. Thank your face for doing such a good job communicating to the world. If you're going to sleep, tell your face its job is over for the day—it's off the clock.

Breathe slowly. Let go of all tension in your temples, eyes, forehead. Feel your forehead melt into the floor as if the weight of your hair is pulling it downwards. Relax your scalp and the crown of your head. Feel them melting into the floor. On each exhalation feel as if gravity is pulling everything toward the floor—upper back and neck, cheeks, ears, and forehead. Just rest.

If you are not going to sleep right now, when you are ready, go on to the rejuvenation exercise.

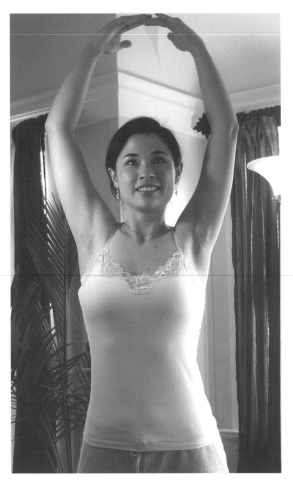

Rejuvenation, Pose 1

Rejuvenation (1)

Open your eyes slowly. Notice the energy bubble shimmering around you. Inhale.

Stretch all your limbs wide, feeling the stretch down to your fingers and toes and far as you can.

Slowly stand up, bringing your head up last.

Lift your arms up in ballerina position around your energy bubble (Pose 1). Feel the bubble expand as you stretch it out with your arms.

Raise your arms to the ceiling and stretch, standing on your tiptoes. Reach towards the ceiling—keep stretching. Feel the bubble burst into a shower of sparkling pinpricks of light all around you. Lower to your heels and, keeping the stretch in your spine, lower your arms and relax your shoulders. You are done!

Note: In times of stress visualize the energy bubble. You will find it helps keep you serene and above the fray.

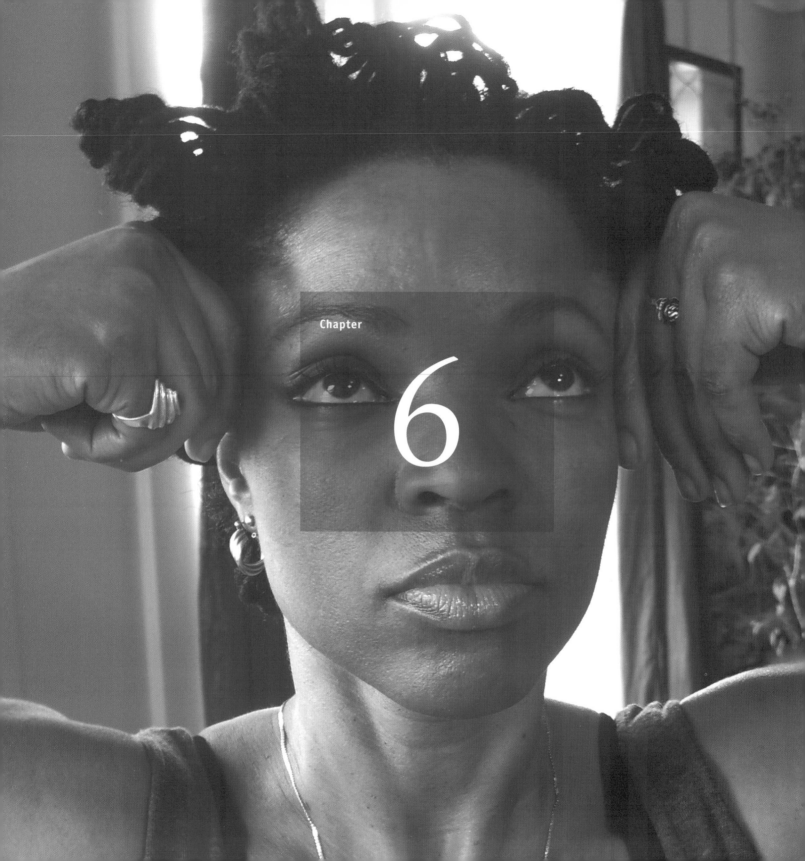

Adding the Power of Belief

"Every French woman dresses as if she is beautiful." —Anonymous

After a bit of practice, you will have acquired reasonable facility with the physical exercises, enough to be able to do them without thinking, because you will have incorporated the memory of how to perform the exercises right into your musculature. You will be able to do them, as they say, in your sleep. Once you have incorporated the physical knowledge of the exercise techniques, you are then free to concentrate on the mental exercises. You are ready for the next step—what I call adding the power of belief.

The Power of Belief

Yoga means "union," and in this part of the exercise routine we take a look at how we can "unionize" the physical face with the inner self in a way that permits our inner being to shine forth, unimpeded by the stresses and worries that tend to contort our features. The face we present to the world will eventually reflect the serenity we feel inside.

The exercise routines I have devised come from a combination of research, study, and practice. The mental techniques that transform simple exercises into a powerful yoga program are drawn from the positive-thinking movement, headed these days by such luminaries as Deepak Chopra and Wayne W. Dyer. The notion that focused intention has the power to get you what you want has many applications. In my case, I intend to use it to transform how we think about beauty and how we regard ourselves when we look in the mirror. From there it's a short hop to transforming how we think and feel about ourselves.

The power to make the change is in your hands. In fact, it's really the heart of the secret. The plastic surgeon can't make you beautiful—it is not in his hands, it is in *yours*. You have the power *within your self*—you just have to know how to tap into it and how to use it.

Here are some techniques to help you get started, but please feel free to revise the language and the structure to suit yourself. The idea is to incorporate the concept of belief into not just your exercises, but also into everything you do. I guarantee you will be overjoyed with the results. Remember the French women who are all dressing as if—act as if, and it will happen.

Don't forget to breathe—and, oh yes, dear students don't ever forget to have fun.

▶ **Week One**

Step One: The Preparation

Look in the mirror. Be objective. Study those areas that need work. Take a picture of yourself and hang it up where you can see it. Write down the areas you are going to concentrate on. Now you are ready to build your own exercise routine.

Step Two: Building an Exercise Routine

After you have practiced all the exercises once or twice you are ready to pick the ones that are most helpful to you. Select the exercises you like from the chart on pages 102-103 and from your short list, come up with your own fifteen-minute routine. You know your own face, you know what areas you want to work on, and after a few attempts you will know which exercises are the most helpful to you.

Do vary the routine a bit, so that once a week you go back and do some exercises not included in your daily routine, just to keep all your muscles in shape. The amount of time you need to devote to your beauty routine, once you've gotten past the preliminary stages, should be about fifteen minutes a day. After two or three months you can shift to the maintenance program, but every once in awhile you should do a longer routine, just to keep in practice.

Group Eight: Forehead and Scalp

Counteracting Horizontal Lines

Scowl Banisher

Group Nine: The Facelift Series

Facelift I

Facelift II

Facelift III

Advanced:
In addition to the beginning exercises, incorporate some of the following exercises for a more challenging routine.

**Group One:
Warm Ups and Stretches**

Arms and Shoulders

Cow Face

Group Three: The Neck

Cow Face for the Neck and Chin

Neck Stretch and Back Bend

Group Five: The Cheeks

Erasing Marionette Lines

**Group Six:
Lips and Mouth**

The Carp Curl—
Advanced

Group Seven: Eyes

Eye Socket Massage and Crow's Feet Extinguisher

For Droopy Eyes

Sample Fifteen-Minute Exercise Routine

Here is a sample exercise routine. This is the one I do when I have time, and it takes me from ten to fifteen minutes.

- **Beginning warm up:**

Bend and Breathe followed by the Spine Stretcher Energizer	2 min.
Circulation: Modified Head Stand	3 min.
Neck: Cow Face for the Neck and Chin	1 min.
Jawline: Jawline Shaper	1 min.
Facelift: Facelift III	1 min.

- *(if I have time I do all three Facelift exercises—these really are my favorite exercises)*

Cheeks: Cheekbone Creator, Erasing Marionette Lines	1 min.
Lips: The Carp Curl	.5 min.
Eyes: Upper Eye, Lower Eye, For Droopy Eyes	2 min.
Forehead: For Horizontal Lines, Scowl Banisher	1.5 min.
Rejuvenation	2 min.

Step Three: Seeing the Results You Want

You are going to see a firmer chin, a younger face, a vibrant, attractive you—whatever is your goal—but make this a goal you can see yourself achieving.

Your goal may sound like a testimonial. For example, "I tried the exercises in *The Yoga Facelift* book and after one week my eyebags were gone and I could see subtle changes taking place in the rest of my face; it was firmer and tauter overall. After three weeks my friends were asking me if I'd had a facelift. After six weeks they were asking for the name of my plastic surgeon. After eight weeks I'd signed a contract with Paramount." You get the picture.

I want you to write your own testimonial tailored to what *you* want to see happen, and you are going to write it *before* you see the results you are raving about. (You can send your testimonial to me after the program works. I'm serious. I expect my mailbox to be overflowing with gladsome tidings.) If you like, you can repeat your goals like mantras as you embark on your self-improvement quest.

Step Four: Getting Excited About It

I learned this part from a psychotherapist in the Bay Area who teaches others how to use visualization techniques with great success. The trick is to visualize the end result that will make you happy and excited and to get excited about it in advance. The simple act of generating enthusiasm about something, as if it has already occurred, alters the energetics of the universal flow in such a way that the power becomes manifest to make the desired result happen. I look at it as a benign game you play with the Universe, in which a *presque* fait accompli becomes a real fait accompli by virtue of a little prestidigitation of the mind, a trompe l'esprit as it were. It's a paradox, but what in the Universe isn't?

One might object that such a practice is just a simple exercise in self-delusion. I have two answers to that. First, so what if it is? If you yourself can't tell the difference between the illusion and the real thing, then it's working for you, and what more do you want? And besides, what isn't illusory anyway?

My second defense addresses that whole pesky "it's all in your mind anyway" business. To my way of thinking, Samuel Johnson destroys the idealist argument, in his inimitable fashion, by kicking a rock and proclaiming "I refute it thusly." If it works, it works, and that's all you need to know. In other words, use objective results, results you can see, to bolster your belief system, and the more positive returns you receive from the external world (and you will receive them) the more your intent will be reinforced. For example, if you visualize a promotion and you get one, it could be a coincidence, but you'd probably keep up the visualization exercises, just in case. In the case of this program you will have a picture that you take of yourself every two weeks and the comments of friends. Believe me, it won't be long before they start noticing.

▶ Weeks Two and Beyond

You are already seeing results. You should take a picture of yourself at the end of week two, again at the end of week four, and yet again at the end of week eight. Compare them and be happy.

You may want to add a mantra to say to the transformed image you see in the mirror. You say this after you are finished with your facial exercises for the day. Here's a suggestion:

I like what see.
I am what I see.
This face is me. I love me.

Repeat this out loud two or three times, or however many times it takes before you feel comfortable saying it. It should feel quite natural, not forced or contrived. Concentrate on the utterance and the conviction behind it with as much attention as you paid to learning the physical exercises. At first it will be just as hard as learning some of the subtler facial movements. As with physical exercise, practice makes perfect. The more you practice, the easier it will become. Give it a try—You have nothing to lose but your wrinkles!

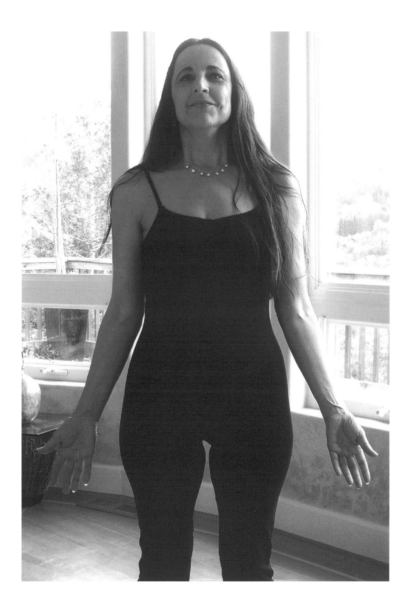

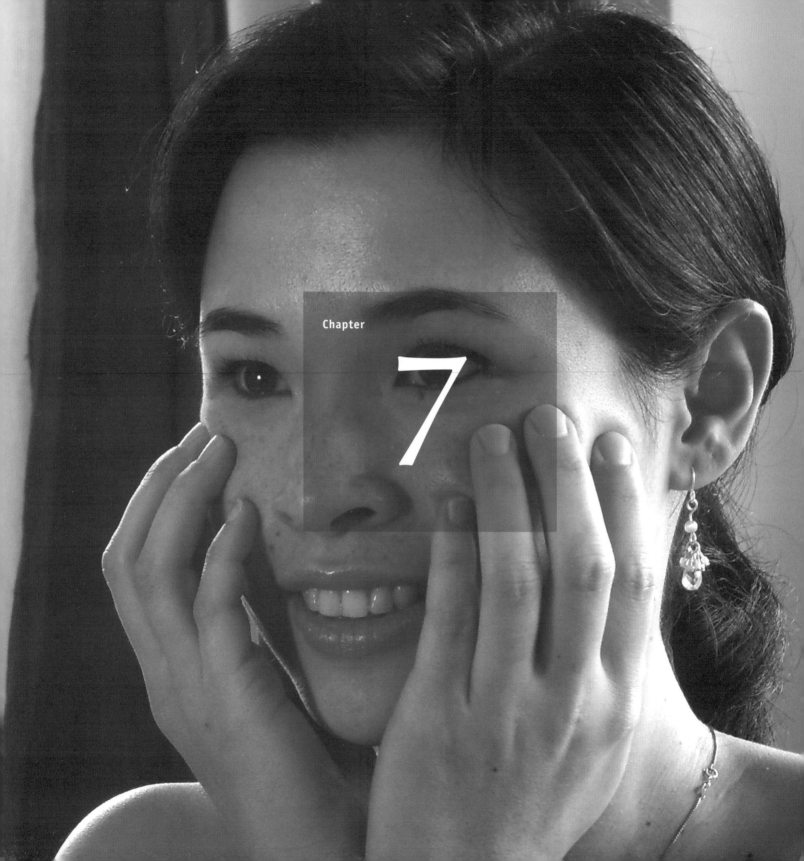

Chapter

7

The Quick Lift

After one to two months of faithfully doing the exercises you chose for your routine in chapter six, you'll be ready for the maintenance program. It will be very helpful for you to have practiced the other exercises in this book before you attempt this one. Once you've had practice exercising individual muscles you are going to find it easy to work the muscles in concert.

The Quick Lift is, as its name suggests, quick and easy. It resembles very much The Lion exercise you learned in chapter two, but with the Quick Lift you are going to exercise the deep muscles of your face without stretching your lips or indeed, moving your face much at all.

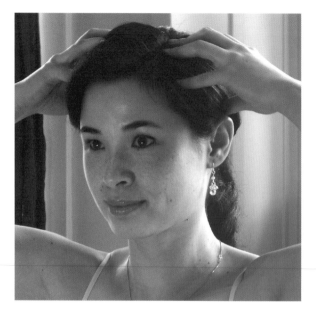

Wake Up, Pose 1

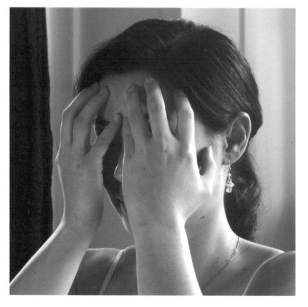

Wake Up, Pose 2

Step One: Focus

Pick a place where you can relax and focus as you do this exercise. I do not recommend doing this in the middle of a traffic jam, for example. Choose a spot where you feel at peace, and if you can, make this "power spot" the place where you always practice the Quick Lift. You will come to regard it as your haven. You may be sitting, standing, or even lying down.

Step Two: Wake Up

Take a deep breath, exhale. Relax. Now we're going to wake up the various muscles in different parts of your face.

1. Place your fingertips on top of your head and, keeping your fingers still, move your head to shift the scalp under them. Feel your scalp muscles move against the pressure of your fingers (Pose 1).

2. Move your fingertips down to your forehead. Now wake up your frontalis muscles by contracting the forehead muscles using your fingertips as resistance (Pose 2).

3. Move your fingertips down to your eye sockets (contracting the orbicularis oculi against the resistance of your fingertips) and effect the same wake-up call (Pose 3).

4. Now move your fingertips down to your cheeks. Contract the cheek muscles against the resistance of your fingertips (Pose 4).

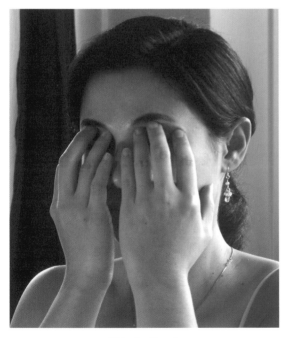

Wake Up, Pose 3

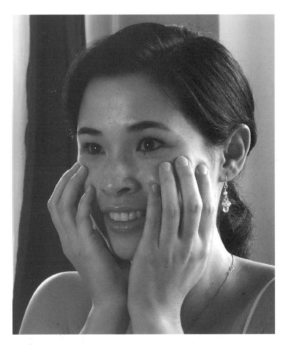

Wake Up, Pose 4

5. Pat your fingertips along your jawline (Pose 5).

6. Brush your fingertips up and down along your neck (Pose 6).

7. Cup your hands gently on your face (Pose 7). By now all the muscles in your scalp, face, and neck should feel tingly and alive.

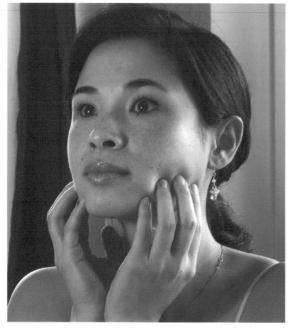

Wake Up, Pose 5

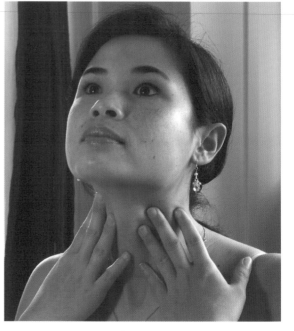

Wake Up, Pose 6

Step Three: Tighten

Remove your hands. Take a deep breath and hold it. Tighten all the muscles of your face and neck. Widen your eyes. Feel your forehead, eye, cheek, lip, jaw, and neck muscles tighten. Hold for ten seconds, working up to thirty seconds as you become more comfortable with the exercise.

Release and exhale. Repeat twice more.

Step Four: Relax

Take several deep breaths. Feel the energy and well-being radiating from your face.

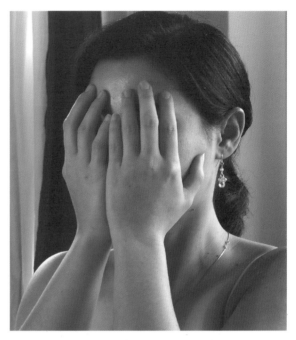

Wake Up, Pose 7

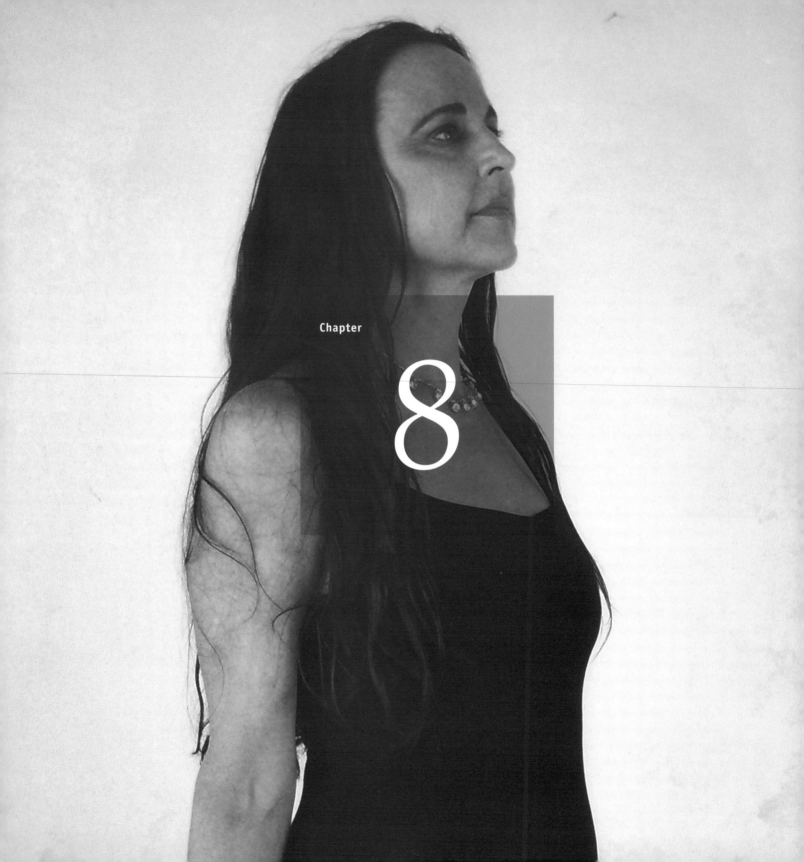

Chapter

8

The Aging Process

Wrinkles, sags, lines, freckles, and liver spots (hyperpigmentation and actinic keratoses, as they are known in the skin trade) are all normal accompaniments of aging—or are they? We hear so much hype about what goes on in the aging process it becomes really difficult to separate fact from fiction. This chapter is a no-nonsense discussion about what we actually know about skin and the aging process. As you have probably guessed by now, aging is more than skin deep.

Before we take a closer look at some of the dynamic processes and mechanisms that contribute to skin aging we need to understand a little bit about that wonderful layer of skin where most of the action is—the dermis.

▶ **The Dermis: An Overview**

The most profound alterations to the skin are actually happening at the dermal rather than the epidermal level. We can describe the dermis as the mattress portion of the skin, and the epidermis as the nice smooth blanket you place on top. Now, what happens to a mattress when its support structure starts to collapse? Of course, it develops sags and creases, and the blanket no longer lies as smoothly on its surface. Wrinkle formation on the skin follows the same procedure, with the epidermis collapsing into the depressions of the uneven dermis.

The dermal layer or extra cellular matrix (ECM) is composed of collagen and elastin fibers and fibroblast cells embedded in a vast array of proteoglycans and other ECM components. Proteoglycans are protein cores to which are attached long chains of repeating disaccharide units. These repeating disaccharide units, called glygosaminoglycans, or GAGs for short, are composed of sugars (glucuronic or iduronic acid) and hexosamines (glucosamine or galactosamine) bound to a protein core. The abundance of hydroxyl, carboxyl, and sulfate groups makes the GAGs intensely hydrophilic (water-loving) and thus able to form porous, hydrated gels. The GAG everyone has heard about is **hyaluronic acid**, a major player in maintaining skin health and beauty.

Skin aging is principally associated with atrophy of the dermal connective tissue. Two related processes contribute to dermal atrophy. The first is **glycation,** which initiates degradation of existing collagen by cross-linking associated with skin wrinkling; the second is skin dehydration due to diminished presence of hyaluronic acid and other GAGs. We need to understand a little bit about these basic processes.

▶ Glycation

Glycation is a normal process and necessary for the correct development of the ECM. However, spontaneous (nonenzymatic) chemical reactions between proteins and sugars can result in the formation of advanced glycation end products, or AGEs (also called Maillard reaction products). These sugar-protein products change progressively to very stable compounds, which form sticky deposits that can accumulate all over the body. They are directly implicated in a variety of ways in the accelerated aging phenomenon. In the dermis, AGEs bridge (cross-link) collagen fibers. In addition, glycation appears to affect the aggregation of collagen monomers into fibers, thus compromising the integrity of the interwoven support structure of the epidermis.

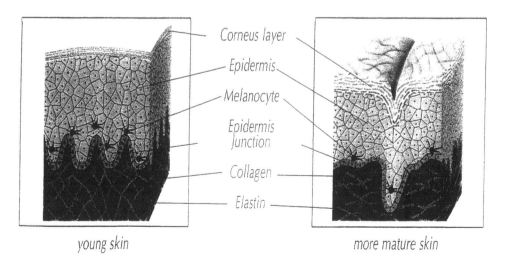

Corneus layer
Epidermis
Melanocyte
Epidermis Junction
Collagen
Elastin

young skin   *more mature skin*

It appears that glycation doesn't influence just the properties of the ECM, but it affects matrix cell interactions as well. Cells grown on matrices composed of glycated proteins differ from normal cells with respect to growth, differentiation, motility, and gene expression. Changes in the ECM and ECM cellular behavior result in the formation of stiff, brittle collagen fibers accompanied by the collapse of dermal supporting structures.

Glycation Inhibition and Glyconutrients

AGEs are irreversible and accumulate as we age, especially in the case of long-lived proteins such as structural collagen. Their role in compromising protein function by contributing to protein cross-linking has consequences for us in the general aging process.

As AGEs have been implicated in such diseases as Alzheimer's, arteriosclerosis, and diabetes. Studies in the fairly recent field of glycobiology suggest that many of these disorders afflicting aging adults can be traced to the lack of an entire category of essential nutrients. The critical missing nutrients are called glyconutrients, and they comprise eight essential carbohydrate monosaccharides. These sugars are crucial for the proper functioning of a huge array of biological processes, from cell building to cell communication. Of the eight carbohydrates essential to proper bodily function, it appears that our modern diets, replete with processed foods, supply us with only two: glucose and galactose. The other six— mannose, fucose, xylose, n-acetyl-glucosamine, n-acetyl-neuramic acid, and n-acetyl-galactosamine—are not commonly found in the modern diet. The consequences of carbohydrate insufficiency have been associated with a vast array of diseases ranging from immune disorders to attention deficit disorder to infections.

I would like to suggest, in addition to all of the preceding, a cosmetic connection—admittedly trivial when stacked up against diabetes and cancer, but nonetheless of concern to all of us faced with the looming prospect of the visible consequences of aging (the appearance of wrinkled, sagging, and dehydrated skin).

It is possible that glyconutrients, by inhibiting AGEs formation, could assist us in delaying the ravages of time, or even help us recapture the supple, unblemished skins we had as children. The research here is sketchy at best, but I suspect we will be hearing more about the glycation process and AGEs as the data comes in. Two areas deserving of further investigation are: (1) skin disorders such as acne vulgaris and psoriasis that are characterized by skin cell overproduction and (2) skin dehydrated due to hyaluronic acid depletion.

▶ Dehydrated Skin and Hyaluronic Acid

Hyaluronic acid is an important component of the ECM, because it is the major water-holding molecule to be found in the connective tissue of the body. One thousand milligrams of hyaluronic acid holds up to six liters of water in the human body. This gel-like disaccharide, composed of alternating molecules of glucosamine and glucuronic acid, is a unique GAG in that it does not contain any sulfate and is not covalently attached to any proteoglycan. This gel-like glycosamineglycans physically supports fibrilar collagen bundles in the dermis.

Hyaluronic acid depletion is one of the primary culprits in dehydrated skin. At around age thirty we start to lose hyaluronic acid at the rate of 1 percent per year. It becomes depleted over time due to age-related slower production rates and oxidative degradation. The production of the disaccharide HA may be stimulated in the presence of adequate amounts of the monosaccharide building blocks needed for its formation. Sufficient amounts of hyaluronic acid in the dermis will keep the collagen scaffold sufficiently hydrated and may also help to prevent the cross-linking of fibers.

▶ Wrinkles, Free Radicals, and Antioxidants

A comprehensive discussion of aging skin must include the free-radical theory of aging, a very important component of an increasingly complicated picture. We have all come to fear the assault of the dreaded free radical—those unstable oxygen molecules that are always in attack mode. To make a long biochemical story short, the theory goes that chronic inflammation caused by free radicals accelerates aging.

The process by which they create wrinkles is complex, but an abbreviated version goes like this: free radicals are released by ultra-violet (UV) exposure (for example) and after a hop, skip, and a jump around various, rather involved biochemical processes they activate production of collagen-digesting enzymes called metalloproteinases. While the function of these metalloproteinases is to remodel sun-injured tissue by manufacturing and reforming collagen, some of these enzymes actually degrade collagen, resulting in an uneven formation of disorganized collagen fibers called solar scars. Repetition of this imperfect building process causes wrinkles.

The oxygen free radical also accounts for diminished amounts of hyaluronic acid in connective tissue throughout the body. The reason there is so much excitement over anti-oxidants these days is that they quench free radicals and thus help prevent oxidative damage.

All of these mechanisms—damaged collagen, collapsing support structure, loss of moisture content, and cell migration—show up in our faces as wrinkled, dry, and sagging skin. The chart below is a simplified version of some of the whys and wherefores of the changes that take place as we age.

Before we take a closer look at some treatments, such as exfoliating peels, we need to talk about one more deep process that explains why our skin, as well as the rest of us, ages.

Problem	Cause(s)	Looks like	Remedies
Diminished moisture content	Diminished hyaluronic acid (HA) production; degradation of HA and other GAGs by free radicals	Dehydration (dry, flaky skin)	Better nutrition; sleep; antioxidant therapy via nutritional supplementation and topical applications
Collapsing support structure	Cross-linking due to glycation; damaged protein accumulation; diminished collagen and elastin production; free radical attacks	Premature wrinkling (from UV exposure and other causes); dynamic wrinkling (expression lines)	Better nutrition; antioxidant supplementation; limit exposure to sun and to chemicals and synthetics in products
Fatty cell migration, decreased muscle tone	Gravity; lack of exercise; lymphatic congestion	Sagging	Exercise, massage, lymphatic drainage
Diminished oil production	Sebaceous gland activity slows down	Dry skin, surface wrinkling	Better nutrition; supplementation with essential fatty acids (EFAs); sleep; moisturizers
Hyperpigmentation	Sun exposure, hormonal changes	Freckles, "sun spots," actinic keratoses	Sun protection, topical skin lighteners

▶ Exfoliation and the Hayflick Limit

Extreme exfoliation treatments such as microdermabrasion, enzyme or AHA peels, Retin-A, and the like are often employed in the antiaging battle. Peels remove the outermost layer of the skin, which stimulates the cells in lower layers to grow and divide, causing the skin to thicken and thus diminishing visible signs of aging. The more you exfoliate, the more cell divisions you have occurring in the lower skin layers.

It is true that exfoliation stimulates cell growth, however, there is one problem: *normal human cells cannot divide indefinitely*. Fibroblasts are a key type of cell in the dermis, important for proper wound repair, collagen production, and epidermal cell replacement. A fibroblast divides about fifty times before it hits the "Hayflick limit." Named after its discoverer, Dr. Leonard Hayflick, the Hayflick limit refers to the number of times a cell divides normally before reaching its senescent stage. Once a cell has reached senescence, division proceeds in a sluggish and inefficient manner, and the cell is unresponsive to various signals from the body. Skin with many senescent cells is usually fragile, blotchy, and easily wrinkled, resembling a plant that slows its leaf and bloom production at the end of its growth cycle. Exfoliation can be a valuable cosmetic tool, but if you overuse it your skin may "hit the Hayflick limit" earlier than it should. In other words, if you increase the frequency of the damage/repair cycle, you could be speeding the cells into senescence and accelerating aging.

In recent years, researchers have discovered the molecular mechanism of the Hayflick limit. (It has to do with the areas at the tips of chromosomes called telomeres.) Medical technologies to eliminate the Hayflick limit may appear at some point in the future, although these advances in technology are likely to work only for those cells whose Hayflick limit has not yet been reached.

An Alternative Beauty Program

We've gone over some of the major causes of skin aging. This was the bad news. But the more we know about causes, the better we can make our remedies. In the next chapter, we embrace the good news—what we can do to slow down the rate at which our skin ages.

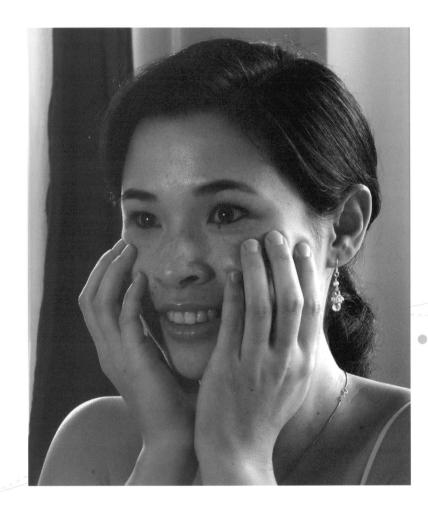

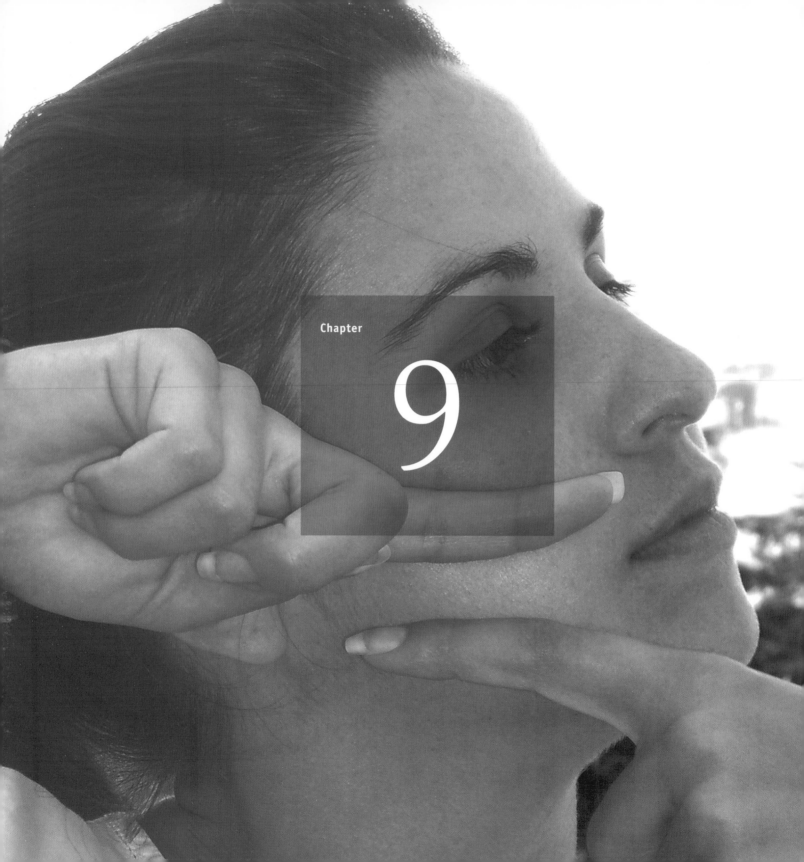

Chapter

9

Beauty Remedies

The whole notion of antiaging has such hostile overtones it's no wonder we regard treatments involving cutting, slashing, burning, paralyzing, or peeling as perfectly normal. But just suppose we take an alternative approach, with the attitude that we should do unto our skin as . . . well, you get the picture. We can start by being kind to our skin—it's a beautiful, intelligent organ that responds almost instantly to gentle treatment. Feed it, nourish it, and above all, love it. Let's look at some practical tips that show us how we can do just that. We're going to talk now about remedies for skin problems, starting with the most important—nutrition.

▶ **Antioxidants and Anti-inflammatories**

It is believed that chronic inflammation caused by free radicals accelerates aging. Part of the free-radical damage related to skin change takes place in the lipid bilayer that makes up the cell plasma membrane. The lipid bilayer maintains the skin's health and beauty by protecting it from external damage and by promoting moisture absorption and retention. Exposure to sun or chemicals activates the enzyme phospholipase A2, which produces arachidonic acid. Activation of the "arachidonic acid cascade" generates inflammatory substances called prostaglandins and leukotrienes. These inflammatory chemicals go on to cause inflammation inside the cell, accelerating its destruction and the aging process in general.

Free radicals are, of course, a natural part of the metabolic process, but emphasizing certain foods in our diet can help to minimize inflammatory cascades. In general, the foods that make up a good diet are whole, enzyme rich, unprocessed, and fresh. Some foods to add, some foods to keep in moderation, and foods to avoid include the following:

Foods to add: apples, burdock, celery, celery root, cold water fish oil and flax seeds (contain omega-3, which quenches the inflammatory cascade), onions (contain high amounts of histamine-quenching quercetin, which inhibits production of leukotrienes), berries (high in bioflavonoids), garlic (rich in sulfur and selenium), cruciferous vegetables (broccoli, cauliflower, cabbage, Brussels sprouts, bok choy, chard, mustard greens, rutabagas, turnips, and kale contain antioxidants), turmeric (contains curcumin, a powerful anti-inflammatory agent excellent for treating inflammatory problems such as arthritis, liver, and gall bladder conditions; curcumin has also been found to block the production of certain prostaglandins and has effects on par with cortisone and nonsteroidal anti-inflammatory drugs but without the side effects).

Foods to keep in moderation: nightshades (tomato, eggplant, peppers, and potatoes contain solamine, a calcium inhibitor), dairy foods except goat- and sheep-milk-based products (contain transfats and animal fats, sources of arachidonic acid), excess salts and sugars (change cell membrane fluidity).

Foods to avoid: highly processed foods and foods containing synthetic colors, flavors, transfats, and/or high-fructose corn syrup.

▶ **Supplements**

- **Essential fatty acids (EFAs):** anti-inflammatory; inhibits arachidonic acid cascades; found in fish, flax, and other omega-3 oils. I recommend 1 teaspoon to 1 tablespoon a day.

- **Bioflavonoids:** found in the white pulpy part of citrus fruit peels; might reduce cuperose when applied topically; quercetin is another good source. Recommendation: 600 to 1200 mg/day, taken internally.

- **Vitamin B complex:** for tissue repair; take 50 mg/day of each B vitamin except for B2, which should not exceed 20 mg/day.

- **Vitamin C:** antioxidant; essential for collagen synthesis; take 3,000 to 6,000 mg/day. (This is a *lot* of vitamin C, and I don't necessarily recommend taking this much all the time. You may do emergency high doses like this when you have a cold or you just want to do some skin repair, but as a daily routine of 1,000 mg—500 mg in the morning and another 500 mg in the evening—is plenty. Large doses won't hurt you, but you may experience diarrhea. If you do, just cut back. We belong to the small set of mammals that doesn't produce their own vitamin C, unfortunately. Goats, for example, produce about 1 gram a day.)

- **Vitamin E:** antioxidant; take 300 to 600 IU/day as mixed tocopherols. Vitamin E mixed tocopherols are considered more bio-useful than alpha-tocopherols alone.

- **Beta-carotene (vitamin A):** known as the skin vitamin; important for new cell growth. There are animal sources (retinol) and vegetable sources (carotenes) in foods. Animal sources are about six times more potent than vegetable sources, but can be toxic if taken in excess. Because of this, vitamin A supplements are restricted to carotenes and limited to under 25,000 IU per pill. Because vitamin A is stored in the liver, it is safer to get your vitamin A in the beta-carotene precursor form, through food sources. Good food sources are fish oil, liver (pork, lamb, chicken, turkey, or beef), eggs, butter, and orange or yellow vegetables or fruits. Broccoli is a good source of vitamin A (green chlorophyll camouflages the yellow carotene color). Another excellent source of both vitamins C and A is the Tibetan goji berry, which are tiny and have the tasty flavor of currants; the dose is 20 to 40 dried berries a day.

- **Bilberry:** enhances the health of capillaries; also a powerful antioxidant. Take 4 to 8 oz of fresh berries, 80 to 160 mg of bilberry extract (25 percent anthocyanidin), or 20 to 40 mg anthocyanosides (powerful antioxidants) daily.

- **Turmeric:** reduces leukotriene formation; increases and potentiates your own cortisol response (cortisol, the so-called "stress' hormone, is involved in skin changes—too little can cause hyperpigmentation, too much may contribute to acne conditions); take 2 to 4 grams three times daily in capsules with equal amounts bromelain; also use in cooking. Turmeric can also be used topically for age or liver spots (see "Alternative Remedies for Common Skin Problems," pages 132-134).

▶ Glycation Inhibition and Glyconutrients

As discussed in the previous chapter, it appears that many of the disorders afflicting aging adults can be traced to the lack of an entire category of essential nutrients. The critical missing nutrients in the new category are called glyconutrients, comprising eight essential carbohydrate monosaccharides. These sugars are crucial for the proper functioning of a huge array of biological processes, from cell building to cell communication.

Sources of glyconutrients are fresh fruits and vegetables, aloe vera juice, Kombucha tea, and human breast milk.

The glyconutritionals are almost impossible to get in the over-processed modern diet. We don't have the variety in our diets that we had as scavengers, and our food is no longer fresh. Look to reputable supplements and never pass up a chance to eat freshly picked or harvested fruits and vegetables.

Let's take a look at a few treatments that draw upon natural sources to address some common problems associated with aging skin.

▶ Acne Rosacea

Rosacea, a problem that has become epidemic among older adults, is related to vascular instability and inflammation. The etiology is unknown. Rosacea can be an annoying, even painful disorder to have, and in the later stages can be very disfiguring, so it is an affliction not to be taken lightly.

Topical Products

Because we absorb at least 60 percent of what we apply to our skins I believe we should take a different perspective on skin products. First, we should never apply anything to our skins that we wouldn't put in our stomachs, and second, we can start looking to skin-care products to do what good food does—that is, they should take care of our skin by providing the specific nutrients this wonderful organ needs to thrive. Nutritional topicals should nourish from the outside in, and in addition, help to heal skin problems and conditions in the same way herbs and vitamin supplements taken internally are intended to do. To my mind, this is a far better approach than slash-and-burn cosmetic intervention, and it is the chief reason I started my own skin-care manufacturing company. I saw the crying need for someone to create topical products that were actually therapeutic—good for you and good for your skin.

Dietary Treatments

The small dietary changes below are worth a try and certainly can't hurt.

1. Because the standard medical approach is to treat rosacea with broad-spectrum antibiotics, one can suspect a relationship to a proliferation of harmful bacteria in the gut. Therefore a good way to treat rosacea internally is to use probiotics to increase quantities of friendly bacteria in the gut. Not too surprisingly, probiotics are also often the best way to treat stubborn cases of cystic acne and acne vulgaris.

2. In addition, it makes sense to try to maintain a diet high in the anti-inflammatory foods discussed previously, since it is highly likely there is a relationship between inflammation and rosacea.

3. Take bioflavonoids to build up your capillaries. To get a great daily dose of bioflavonoids eat 4 to 8 oz of fresh bilberries and 80 to 160 mg of bilberry extract (25 percent anthocyanidin) or 20 to 40 mg anthocyanosides daily.

Topical Treatments

Some topical treatments include:

- **Cleansing:** with whole milk yogurt (contains acidophilus, a friendly bacteria) twice a day.

- **Masks:** use yogurt, or a combination of yogurt and honey (which is a humectant, antiviral, and antimicrobial). Colloidal oatmeal and/or crushed berries can also be added to the above masks (see "Bioflavonoids" page 134).

- **Sunscreen:** use daily, even when it's cloudy, as you need protection against the UVA rays (out from dawn to dusk) that can trigger inflammation. Use only mineral (titanium dioxide and zinc oxide) sunscreens; this is very important, because chemical sunscreens can be extremely irritating to rosacea sufferers. Look especially for zinc oxide, which is a good anti-inflammatory, very healing, and provides the broadest, full-spectrum protection available. (Marie-Véronique Crème de Jour [SPF 15 or 25+] is a sunblock specifically designed for rosacea sufferers. It contains natural sunscreen agents like zinc oxide, emu oil, and red raspberry oil, which are also highly anti-inflammatory.)

About Ultraviolet Waves

Ultraviolet (UV) light has shorter wavelengths than visible light. There are three types of ultraviolet rays that should concern us when we think about sun protection. UVC rays are the shortest of the three types, with wavelengths less than 280 nm (nanometers). Short wavelength, high-energy UVC rays are implicated in skin cancers, particularly basal cell carcinomas. These rays are ordinarily completely absorbed by the ozone layer; however, as this protective shield thins or is even, as in some areas of the world like Australia, nonexistent, we are more at risk of exposure to these damaging rays. UVB rays, the burning rays, range from 280- to 320-nm on the spectrum. The SPF (sun protection factor) rating by FDA regulation need only apply to UVB rays. Look at the label on your sunblock to make sure it provides both UVB and UVA protection. Long-wave UVA rays are in the 320- to 400-nm range. UVA or "wrinkling" rays, present from sunup to sundown, can penetrate clouds and glass. Protection should be year-round, not just when the sun is out. When looking for effective sun protection, bear in mind that zinc oxide offers full-spectrum UVA protection, up to 400 nm, while titanium dioxide blocks UVA rays only up to 350- to 360-nm.

133

An easy mnemonic for remembering the effect of each type of UV ray is:

C = cancer,   **B** = burning,   **A** = aging

- **Topical anti-inflammatories:** such as emu oil, zinc oxide, turmeric, raspberry seed oil, colloidal oatmeal, seaweed, arnica, and sea buck-thorn oil.

- **Bioflavonoids:** those in berries and the white pulpy part of citrus skins may help with cuperose, or dilated capillaries. Eat the fruit often and don't forget to make a mask with the berries and/or the citrus pulp. Raspberry seed oil is also high in bioflavonoids.

▶ Liver Spots

Liver spots, also known as age spots, are yellowish brown flat spots that look like large freckles. They are thought to be caused by aging, too much sun, impaired liver function, and a dietary or nutritional deficiency. (Note: If you have irregular, dark spots that increase in size or change color or texture, have them checked by a doctor.) As we age, our metabolism changes, and the liver may become so overwhelmed with toxins that it cannot rid the body of them. Oxidation within the body and the lack of antioxidants also plays an important role in this process.

Dietary Treatment

Take 2 to 4 grams of turmeric three times daily in capsules with equal amounts bromelain.

Topical Treatment

Mix 1 teaspoon tomato juice and 1/2 teaspoon lemon juice, then add enough organic turmeric to make a paste. Apply to spots twice daily.

▶ Actinic keratoses

Actinic keratoses are the raised spots, usually dark brown in color, that are presumed to be caused by sun (actinic) exposure. Again, antioxidants play an important role in preventing their appearance.

Topical Treatment

Add 1 clove pressed garlic and a pinch of tumeric to 6 teaspoons aloe vera gel. Apply to spots at night.

▶ Seborrheic keratoses

These yellow or brown oval spots with clear perimeters and raised surfaces develop in middle age and are enhanced by sun exposure. They can be treated in the same manner described for actinic keratoses.

▶ Hyperpigmentation

Hyperpigmentation is linked to sun damage, but other factors can contribute to it, including diminished cortisol production (associated with Addison's disease), over-secretion of cortisol brought about by stress, hormonal changes, and post-inflammatory response (from injury or infection).

Dietary Treatment

Taking turmeric may help as it potentiates cortisol. Take 2 to 4 grams three times daily in capsules with equal amounts bromelain.

Topical Treatments

- **Cleansing:** with yogurt or a milk product containing lactic acid helps to whiten the skin.

- **Masks:** (1) Make a paste by mixing colloidal oatmeal and turmeric with water, milk, whipped cream, or yogurt. Apply and leave on thirty to forty minutes. (2) Spread a thin layer of olive oil on the face, avoiding the eye area. Cut a fresh lemon into quarters, then rub one quarter of the lemon over your face for twenty to thirty seconds. Rinse with cool water.

(3) Purée a two-inch slice of fresh cucumber, 1 teaspoon lemon juice, and 2 tablespoons cream or plain yogurt in a blender. Apply mixture to face, avoiding the eye area. Allow thirty minutes to dry. Rinse with cool water.

- **Skin bleaching agents:** lemon, pearl powder, grated raw potato (contains calecholase, a natural skin lightener), zinc oxide, licorice root, green tea, yellow dock, lactic acid.

- **Avoid:** products containing hydroquinone, which is banned in most countries as it has been charged with causing cell mutations and is considered site toxic to cells. Uva ursi, or bearberry, contains hydroquinone and should probably be avoided. Essential oils in the citrus family, bergamot essential oil, retinoic acid, Retin-A or Renova, fragrances, and alcohol can create photosensitivity and increase hyperpigmentation, so they should not be applied externally.

> **For Dark Circles Under the Eyes**
>
> Do this when you have ten to twenty minutes of free time to just relax. Cut out two pieces of cheesecloth big enough to hold 2 to 3 tablespoons of grated potato. Grate a raw, white potato, then wrap the potato in the pieces of cheesecloth. Make two "potato wraps." Place one potato wrap on each eye so that the juice seeps onto the undereye area. Lie back and enjoy for ten to fifteen minutes.

▶ Wrinkles

Dietary Treatment

Remember, there is an important connection between inadequate nutrition and wrinkle formation. Vitamin C is absolutely essential, not just as an antioxidant, but also because it is absolutely crucial to one stage of the collagen biosynthesis process. Without vitamin C you do not make new collagen. The glyconutritonals that inhibit glycation (which leads to cross-linking and brittle collagen fibers) are also important to add to your diet; the best sources are homegrown fruits and vegetables that you pick and eat right away. (Glyconutritionals are in all the Marie-Véronique topical products, so that's another way you can get a dose for your skin. Please see the last chapter for further discussion.)

Topical Treatments

Feeding your face from the outside will nourish and hydrate your skin and help to soften wrinkles. Here are a few things you can do. Note: If you have a garden, use your imagination—almost anything that you can eat raw, or prepare for eating by cooking, can go on your face.

- **Cleansing and masks for exfoliation:** I've discussed my stand on extreme exfoliation in chapter eight; I do believe that microdermabrasion, Retin-A, glycolic acid peels, and so on ultimately accelerate aging and should be avoided. Exfoliation treatments have achieved great popularity because they act like a quick fix—removing the top layer of the epidermis does give a temporary rosy blush to the skin. However, in the interests of preserving the skin over the long haul, I suggest exfoliating gently with natural food products. You will ultimately get the same beautiful results, but without damaging your skin.

- **Alpha-hydroxy acids (AHAs) and enzymes:** There are two AHAs that are safe to use when you get them from food: citric acid and lactic acid. Buttermilk, yogurt, or sour cream contain lactic acid, which helps the biosynthesis of glycosaminoglycans and leaves your skin feeling soft and supple. You can cleanse with them, or apply them as a mask, leaving them on for twenty to thirty minutes. The citric acid in lemon juice makes a great mask as well. I suggest applying a thin layer of olive oil over the skin, then rubbing the juice from a quarter of a fresh lemon over the olive oil. Leave on for thirty seconds or so, then rinse. Papaya makes a great enzyme mask, but don't leave it on longer than ten minutes. Remember to wear your sunscreen after any kind of exfoliation treatment, as you will have compromised the stratum corneum, your environmental protective barrier. External nourishment is more important than exfoliation, which is overrated as a wrinkle fighter in my estimation. If you feel the need to use AHAs other than lactic acid, it's a good idea to vary AHA treatments with nourishing masks (made with honey, oatmeal, or avocado to name just a few) to avoid thinning the skin.

- **Hydrating, nourishing masks:** Make carrot juice, drink it, and use the pulp for a mask. Leave on for thirty to forty minutes. You can add honey, yogurt, or seaweed. Seaweed is an excellent moisturizer that increases circulation, helps eliminate toxins, and delivers nutrients and minerals to the cells.

- **Vitamin C:** Yes, it can be applied topically, but be careful how you do it. Most vitamin C in creams and lotions have already oxidized (that's why vitamin C is a good antioxidant!), and the lotion may actually release free radicals on the skin when applied. Best to get stable, phyto-based sources of vitamin C or use fresh fruits, such as citrus and berries. The vitamin C in the citrus pulp and berries will build collagen and help in cellular repair, while the bioflavonoids will help strengthen capillaries.

- **Sun protection:** UV protection is a full-time affair, since the wrinkling UVA rays are present from dawn to dusk, rain or shine. Use a mineral sunscreen. Wear a hat. Try to avoid exposure from 10 A.M. to 2 P.M., the burning time. Remember that UVA rays reflect from shiny surfaces, so your exposure is greatly increased in traffic, at the beach, or on the ski slopes.

- **Hyaluronic acid:** After age thirty, we lose approximately 1 percent hyaluronic acid per year. You can take hyaluronic acid supplements, but it will go to your joints and not your skin. Applied topically? The hyaluronic acid molecule is very large and probably does not absorb well. Because it is a disaccharide composed of glucuronic acid and glucosamine, adding the glyconutritionals to your diet will help your body produce more hyaluronic acid. (If you are looking for a topical treatment, the Marie-Véronique Skin Therapy company has developed a new product called Renaissance, which consists of all the saccharides your skin needs to biosynthesize hyaluronic acid in a form that ensures penetration to the dermis.)

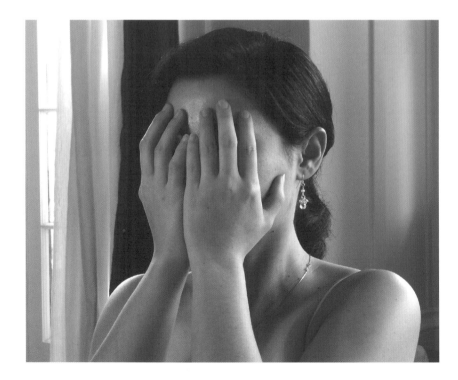

▶ DMAE

DMAE, short for dimethylaminoethanol, is a naturally occurring substance that facilitates the synthesis of the neurotransmitter acetylcholine. DMAE also may stimulate the synthesis of phosphatidylcholine, an important component of cell membranes. (In fact, DMAE is far better known and researched as a "smart drug" than a skin-firming agent. In a number of studies DMAE has been shown to reduce age-related decline in cognitive ability and memory.)

It has been demonstrated that DMAE causes some degree of skin tightening, most probably by boosting acetylcholine, the neurotransmitter that sends the message to the muscles to contract. If the effects of DMAE taken by itself are noticeable, think how much more dramatic the results will be by adding mild facial exercises to the program. In that case, you will be contracting muscles voluntarily to achieve a youthful, toned look to the face and neck.

▶ Facial Sculpting and Lymphatic Drainage

One physical law we'd all prefer to break but unfortunately can't is the law of gravity. At a certain age everything in our bodies start to go south—and as the fatty cells start their downward migration the effects on the face and neck are quite noticeable. A Bay Area practitioner and friend, Colette DeVore, LAc, MS, TCM (traditional Chinese medicine), has developed a massage technique called facial sculpting, which addresses sagging muscles. She moves the muscles of the face back to where they were before they sagged over the years, which results in a dramatically lifted look. To address a sagging muscle, you might go with the formula: get it up with facial sculpting, and keep it up with exercise!

In conjunction with facial sculpting, lymphatic drainage reduces fluid in the face. Fluid accounts for a great deal of sagging tissue over time. To drain fluid from your face, simply lay two fingers under your cheekbone where the fluid accumulates (Pose 1) and with the bottom finger push, with a steady gentle motion, down your neck and into the hollow above your collarbone (Pose 2).

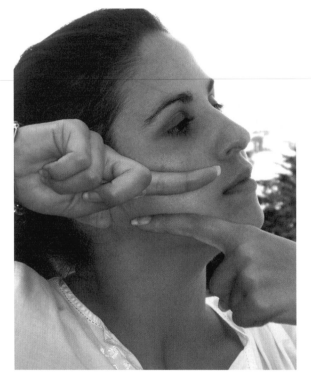

Lymphatic Drainage, Pose 1

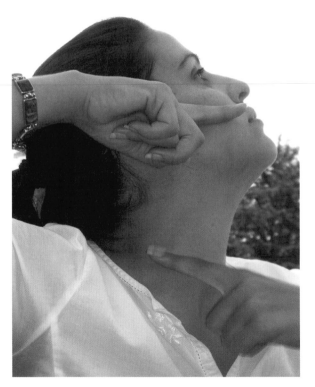

Lymphatic Drainage, Pose 2

▶ Sleep

To paraphrase the great Edward Devere (who some people know as Shakespeare, but that's another story), "Sleep knits up the raveled skin and makes us fair"—uh, well, you get the idea. The most important hours for sleep occur between 10 P.M. and 3 A.M.. This is when melatonin, the great antioxidant, makes its rounds throughout the body, scooping up free radicals and repairing damage. No sleep, no skin repair, and we all know what that looks like.

▶ Water

The controversy rages around water—especially how much to drink. Rather than engage in that debate I prefer to add my own two cents' worth. Remember hyaluronic acid, that wonderful substance that gives our skin tissue that childlike, plump look? Because of its disaccharide components, hyaluronic acid is extremely hydrophilic—it has a great ability to bind water. When we drink water we want to be able to do the same thing—that is, bind water to systems so it can truly hydrate our tissues. My suggestion is to add to one glass of your water (perhaps the first glass of the morning) a bit of aloe vera juice. Aloe vera is high in mucopolysaccharides that will help you bind water to your system.

Also remember that we get a lot of water from the food we eat, especially fruit. As far as I'm concerned, a slice of watermelon ought to count as one glass of water—it is 98 percent water, and the 2 percent sugar content helps bind all that water so that you are actually utilizing it instead of excreting it (along with all the vitamins and minerals you've been taking such pains to ingest).

Chapter

10

Marie-Véronique Skin Therapy

The Birth of a Company

I am a self-confessed skin-care junkie. This was fine when I worked in information technology as a technical writer and had the resources to support my habit. While I managed a brave grin into my bathroom mirror each morning, the shelves in the cabinet on the other side were groaning under the weight of all my antiaging creams, worth their weight in gold, or in some cases platinum. Then the tech industry's bubble burst, and, hunched under the dark cloud of many months of unemployment, I finally had to quit my addiction to antiaging agents cold turkey. It turned out to be a blessing in disguise, as those things often are. The silver lining to the dark cloud was the realization that most of those overpriced goos I was using were drying out my skin, exacerbating my rosacea, or giving me rashes. When I went back to school and got my aesthetician's license, I began to figure out why they weren't living up to all the promises they were making.

Armed with what I like to call "a license to peel," I started working at the Elephant Pharmacy in Berkeley, California. I came aboard on the day of the store's grand opening, in fact, and we're still going strong. It's the ideal environment for me. Surrounded by skilled practitioners of alternative healing methods such as herbology, naturopathy, homeopathy, and Ayurvedic and Chinese medicine, I was able to see how their ancient techniques could be adapted to and complement the kind of skin care I wanted to deliver. True and lasting skin care, I came to be aware, is a holistic science, and you create an even more powerful therapy when you address aging from the inside out as well as from the outside in. It became obvious to me that nutrition was a big part of skin care, so I began making diet and digestion a regular part of my consultations. I learned a lot from my early client sessions. It didn't take long for me to realize that digestive problems and acne rosacea (as well as acne vulgaris) tended to go hand in hand. I am convinced that no program that claims to control these disorders can do so without looking at the dietary component.

Gradually I began to see where my strengths were and what my specialties would become. I wanted to treat mature skin and acne rosacea, categories that often overlap as rosacea usually afflicts people from age thirty-five and up. I learned that nutrition was one way to improve skin condition, but was there anything else I could do? Indeed there was. I began a serious inquiry into the reputed benefits of topically applied products. As I soon discovered, the downside of product use ranged from an exacerbation of problems to allergic reactions. I also took issue with the shameless fashion with which some companies were routinely picking our pockets. For example, one famous company charges $125 an ounce for an eye cream whose main ingredient is hydrogenated vegetable oil. If you like the feel of trans fats on your skin, I suggest going straight for the cheaper Crisco. Please understand that while neither product has my recommendation, I believe you'll not only save money using solid vegetable oil, but you'll also be safer, as it doesn't contain all the preservatives, fillers, and fragrances found in the eye cream.

The eye cream story reminds me that a big part of my job is informing the public. I'll collar anyone who will listen and tell them that we absorb approximately 60 percent of what we put on our skins, and that we need to be as vigilant about what we put *on* our bodies as what we put *in* them.

Skin-care products on the department store and pharmacy shelves continue to multiply like Wal-Marts. In addition to their bunnylike reproductive capacities it seemed they all had a proclivity for making unsubstantiated claims, such as "cures rosacea," "banishes wrinkles," or "rejuvenates." We've heard them all, and you probably all know from experience, just as I do, that they don't live up to their claims.

My frustration with the ersatz ingredients and overpriced, corporate-sponsored skin creams motivated me to create my own line of skin-care products, which I call Marie-Véronique Skin Therapy. I believe my products are the very first and best lotions and creams to deliver clinically proven nutritional supplements—including glyconutrients and antioxidants—transdermally. Good for the skin is good for the body, and the feedback I began to get from my customers in terms of the results has been nothing short of phenomenal. If you care to see some of these testimonials or read more about the products I invite you to go to *www.organicskintherapy.com*. Bottom line? My stuff simply works. Voila!

I know Berkeley folks will understand what I mean when I say my goal has been to do for the skin-care industry what Alice Waters has done for gourmet cooking. Until she came along we thought it was normal for food to have artificial colors and flavor enhancers. In the fifties I grew up on red Jets cereal and blue Popsicles. As kids we thought real food was supposed to taste super sweet, have a rubbery texture, glow with vibrant Crayola colors, and last forever in the cupboard. Some of the tastiest morsels even had their own special geometry—from triangles, swirls, and pillows to horns, horses, and hockey pucks.

Thanks to Alice we are now aware that truly healthy and flavorful food doesn't come out of boxes endorsed by cartoon characters. We've figured out that organic ingredients, freshly prepared, make for delicious eating that is also nutritional. Now those of us who are making nouvelle cuisine products for the skin are seeing how the same culinary standards that apply to freshly prepared organic ingredients can become topically applied products that are just as good for you. And *because* they are intrinsically good for you, my products *do*, in fact, work! Surprising as it may seem, this news comes as quite a revelation in the skin-care world. *Merci beaucoup*, Alice Waters.

Marie-Véronique Products

I make products that are all natural and organic. They contain optimum amounts of nutritional ingredients (including phyto-based antioxidants and glyconutritionals) and minimal amounts of preservatives. In fact, my online organic products are just like the best food you can buy: they are made fresh, in small batches; nourish from the outside in with bioactive, nutritional ingredients; and have no synthetic preservatives. I believe outside-in nourishment is especially helpful as we age and our digestive systems are not as efficient as they once were. I feel enough like a skin-care cop whose duty it is to protect the public from predatory practices that I am tempted to borrow from the police department's motto—"Marie-Véronique Skin Therapy: To Nourish and Protect."

▶ Nourishment

Every product in the Marie-Vèronique line contains the monosaccharide complex that provides the missing six carbohydrates. In addition, we know we need to get as many antioxidants as possible into our systems every day, and plant-based supplements are vastly superior to their synthetic counterparts in providing effective antioxidant protection. Marie-Vèronique products contain a phyto-based antioxidant complex composed of mixed tocopherol vitamin E, quercetin, grape-skin extract, green-tea extract, and the Australian bush plant.

▶ Protection

The primary cause of skin aging is UV exposure. Most sunscreens contain phenobenzones and/or octyl methoxycinnimate, which may irritate skin. The Marie-Véronique Crème de Jour is unique in the field of UV protectors in that it contains a full range of sunblocks, *all* of which are natural. In addition to having full-spectrum UVA and UVB protection with zinc oxide, it has natural moisturizing UV blocking agents: emu oil (great for wrinkles and scar tissue), pearl powder (a whitening agent), shea butter, cocoa butter, coconut oil, and green tea.

The Titanium Dioxide Controversy

I have recently phased out the use of titanium dioxide in my sunblock since it is not known at this time whether titanium oxide is truly an inert mineral, especially when it is dispersed in small particles. Many companies are using micronized versions of titanium dioxide and zinc oxide, but small particle behavior (at sizes under 50 microns, say) is unpredictable. Zinc oxide (not micronized) provides full-spectrum UVA/UVB protection and is anti-inflammatory. When combined with the other natural sunscreen agents mentioned previously, it makes for a truly comprehensive and effective formulation.

For a detailed list of the products in the Marie-Véronique Skin Therapy line, including ingredients and directions for use, please consult the Appendix at the back of this book.

To learn more about titanium dioxide please visit *http://www.organicskintherapy.com/titanium_dioxide.html*.

Reformulating the Equation

A customer of mine by the name of Miranda recently asked me, "Why are you doing all this?"—meaning developing products, promoting massage techniques, teaching classes, and now writing this book. I hope my reply did not make her eyes glaze over, but the subject of beauty is anything but trivial.

A partial answer may lie in the source of our desire to attract. This natural and human desire is linked to the urge to reproduce, and since youth broadcasts fecundity, we can see where the youth equals beauty equation comes from. This is our hardwiring dictating the rules of the game.

But consider this: in an overpopulated world, nonfecundity should have its attractions, not to mention its attractors. And by now we've all had decades to develop replacement allures. Whether it is interesting conversation, mastery of the unicycle, or inventing a fantastic goat cheesecake, whatever we've taken the trouble to learn, to master, or to wield is certain to fascinate someone out there somewhere. Growing older is wonderful—when we reach a certain age we can finally throw off the shackles of biological hardwiring.

But the real attraction at any age is good health, and so, drawing a deep breath, I said to Miranda that I would like to change the equation to read health equals beauty rather than youth equals beauty.

She responded that indeed, we are hardwired to want to be attractive, but there is something else going on—there is an aesthetic need that we fulfill when we look in a mirror and like what we see. We are visual beasts, we like—no, we need—to look around us and see beauty, and that same intrinsic need operates when we look at ourselves. I think she's right. And so, for the Mirandas of this, our brave new world in the making, I write this book, dedicated to helping us all find a way to like what we see.

Appendix

My line of Marie-Véronique Skin Therapy products includes the following lotions and sprays. Directions for use as part of your Yoga Facelift regimen are also included here.

Crème de Nuit: For dry, mature skins. Herbal and white-tea infused spring water (aqua), calendula-infused Simmondsia Chinensis (jojoba) Oil, Persea Gratissima (avocado) oil, Oryza Sativa (rice) bran oil, Triticum Vulgate (wheat germ) oil, Prunus Armeniaca (apricot) kernel oil, Butyrospermum parkii (shea butter), Cocus Nucifera (coconut) oil, Borago officinalis (borage) oil, Oenothera Biennis (evening primrose) oil, Rubus idaeus (red raspberry) seed oil, vaccinium oxycoccos (cranberry) seed oil, Hippophae rhamnoides (sea buckthorn) oil, Theoboma cacao (cocoa) seed butter, Rosa Damascena (rose) hydrosol, Fucus Vesiculosis (seaweed) extract, vegetable emulsifying wax, lecithin, Panax ginseng, allantoin, gingko biloba, alpha-lipoic acid, DMAE, tocopherol (Vitamin E), potassium sorbate, quercetin, Carnellia synensis (green tea) extract, resveratrol (grape skin) extract, Australian Bush plum (plant-based Vitamin C), Aloe Barbadensis (aloe) extract, gum ghatti, xantham gum, gum tragacanth, acai powder, camu camu powder, Rosa rubiginosa (rosehip seed) essential oil, daucus carota sativa (carrot seed) essential oil, cistus (rockrose) essential oil, Helichryssum (everlasting) essential oil

Directions: Pump small amount into palm of hand, rub hands together, then apply gently to face with patting motions. Do not use around eyes. Use nightly after cleansing.

Crème de Jour 15: for all skin types, including but not limited to: sensitive, allergenic, rosacea-prone. Herbal and white-tea infused spring water (aqua), calendula-infused Simmondsia Chinensis (jojoba) oil, Persea Gratissima (avocado) oil, emu oil, Limnanthes alba (meadowfoam seed) oil, Triticum Vulgate (wheat germ) oil, Cocus Nucifera (cocunut) oil, Rubus idaeus (red raspberry) seed oil, vaccinium oxycoccos (cranberry) seed oil, Hippophae rhamnoides (sea buckthorn) oil, Butyrospermum parkii (shea butter), Theoboma cacao (cocoa) seed butter, zinc oxide, pearl powder, Rosa Damascena (rose) hydrosol, Fucus Vesiculosis (seaweed) extract, allantoin, Panax ginseng, vegetable emulsifying wax NF, lecithin, tocopherol (Vitamin E), potassium sorbate, quercetin, Carnellia synensis (green tea) extract, resveratrol (grape skin) extract, Australian Bush plum (plant-based Vitamin C), Aloe Barbadensis (aloe) extract, gum ghatti, xantham gum, gum tragacanth, acai powder, camu camu powder, Rosa rubiginosa (rosehip seed) essential oil, daucus carota sativa (carrot seed) essential oil, Helichryssum (everlasting) essential oil

Crème de Jour 25+: contains double concentrations of sunblock agents zinc oxide

Directions: Pump small amount into palm of hand, rub hands together, then apply gently to face with patting motions. Smooth on a second layer and rub into face, concentrating on exposed areas in cases where extra protection is needed. May be used around eyes. Use daily after cleansing.

Serumdipity: for dry skin. Great for wrinkles, scars, and stretch marks. Calendula-infused Simmondsia Chinensis (jojoba) oil, emu oil, Borago officinalis (borage) oil, Oenothera Biennis (evening primrose) oil, Rubus idaeus (red raspberry) seed oil, vaccinium oxycoccos (cranberry) seed oil, Hippophae rhamnoides (sea buckthorn) oil, Tamanu oil, squalane, Rosa Cunina (rosehip) oil, tocopherol (Vitamin E), daucus carota sativa (carrot seed) essential oil, Helichryssum (everlasting) essential oil, rose essential oil, frankincense essential oil

Serumdipity: for oily, break-out prone skin. Calendula-infused Simmondsia Chinensis (jojoba) Oil, emu oil, Borago officinalis (borage) oil, Oenothera Biennis (evening primrose) oil, Rubus idaeus (red raspberry) seed oil, vaccinium oxycoccos (cranberry) seed oil, Hippophae rhamnoides (sea buckthorn) oil, Tamanu oil, squalane, Rosa Cunina (rosehip) oil, tocopherol (Vitamin E), daucus carota sativa (carrot seed) essential oil, Helichryssum (everlasting) essential oil, palmarosa essential oil, lavender essential oil, German chamomile essential oil

Directions: massage into face and neck. For oily skin or skin prone to break outs use instead of a nightly cream-based moisturizer. Dry skin: at night, apply to face and neck, concentrating on dry patches. Follow with Crème de Nuit or other moisturizer. Special uses: may be used to soften scars and stretch marks and to soothe eczema.

Celtic Rain Hydrating Mist: for all skin types. Carnellia synensis (green tea) infusion, Aloe Barbadensis (aloe) gel, arabinogalactan, Oryza sativa (rice) starch, gum ghatti, glucosamine Hcl, gum tragacanth, Daucus Carota sativa (carrot seed) essential oil

Directions: After cleansing, mist on face to hydrate and nourish. Use whenever extra hydration is needed.

Affirmatif Facial Firming Spray: for all skin types. Carnellia synensis (green tea) infusion, Aloe Barbadensis (aloe) gel, arabinogalactan, Oryza sativa (rice) starch, gum ghatti, glucosamine Hcl, gum tragacanth, DMAE, pearl powder, Panax ginseng, Daucus Carota sativa (carrot seed) essential oil, cistus (rockrose) essential oil, Green myrtle essential oil, rose essential oil

La Vie en Rose Mask: for oily and problem skin. Colloidal oatmeal, adzuki bean powder, rice bran powder, marshmallow root powder, rose petal powder, rose clay, Norwegian kelp powder, dulse powder, green-blue algae, turmeric

Directions: Mix 1 tsp of powder with yoghurt, water, or cream to make a thin paste. Apply to skin, leave on for 20-30 minutes. Rinse thoroughly. Use 1-2 times a week.

Oil-Free Oatmeal Honey Cleanser: for sensitive, dry skin. *Carnellia synensis (green tea) infusion, Citrus Aurantium Dulcis (neroli) hydrosol, Aloe Barbadensis (aloe) gel, colloidal oatmeal, raw honey, carageenan (irish moss), xantham gum, Palmaria Palmata (dulse), Oryza sativa (rice) starch, Ascophyllum nodosum (kelp), marshmallow root powder, blue-green algae, Lavandula argustifloria (lavender) essential oil, Pelargonium grareolens (geranium) essential oil*

Oatmeal Honey Scrub: for normal to oily skin. *Carnellia synensis (green tea) infusion, Citrus Aurantium Dulcis (neroli) hydrosol, Aloe Barbadensis (aloe) gel, colloidal oatmeal, raw honey, carageenan (irish moss), xantham gum, Palmaria Palmata (dulse), Oryza sativa (rice) starch, Ascophyllum nodosum (kelp), marshmallow root powder, blue-green algae, jojoba wax beads, Lavandula argustifloria (lavender) essential oil, Pelargonium grareolens (geranium) essential oil, Peppermint essential oil*

Renaissance: for skin renewal. A lotion designed to replenish, nourish, and rejuvenate, it is excellent for skin renewal and addressing skin problems such as rosacea and wrinkles. glyconutrients: arabinogalactan, glucosamine HCl, gum tragacanth glucuronic acid. *other: glycosamino-glycans, lactic acid, anti-inflammatories, antioxidants, IGF-1 (Insulin-like growth factor-1), astragalus, aloe vera, green tea, bioflavonoids, essential fatty acids omega-3, 6, 7, liposomes. essential oils: helichryssum*

Renaissance Ultra: for lightening skin. Recommended for hyperpig-mentation. glyconutrients: arabinogalactan, glucosamine HCl, gum tragacanth glucuronic acid. *other: glycosaminoglycans, lactic acid, anti-inflammatories, antioxidants, IGF-1 (Insulin like growth factor-1),*

astragalus, aloe vera, green tea, bioflavonoids, essential fatty acids omega-3, 6, 7, liposomes, uva ursi, pearl powder, licorice root essential oils: helichryssum

Directions: Use in the morning and the evening after cleansing. Fill the dropper with lotion and squeeze into the palm of your hand. Spread the lotion in a *thin* layer over the entire face and neck. One half ounce should last about four weeks. You may use it under the eyes. Let dry for about five minutes, then apply Creme de Nuit or Creme de Jour as usual. To increase its efficacy, drink a glass of water with each application. The lotion has hydrophillic properties that will help you bind the water molecule at the dermal level. *Keep refrigerated.*

(For more information about Renaissance please go to: www.organicskintherapy.com/renaissance.html)

Suggested Daily Skin Care Regimen

Day	Night
Wash with cleanser or scrub	Wash with cleanser or scrub
Mist with Celtic Rain	Mist with Celtic Rain
Apply Crème de Jour	Massage with Serumdipity if skin is very dry
Pat eye candy under eyes	Apply Crème de Nuit
optional: apply Renaissance, let dry about five minutes, apply Crème de Jour	**optional:** apply Renaissance after Serumdipty, let dry five minutes, apply Crème de Nuit

Mature skins, hyperpigmented skins or skins with a tendency to rosacea: Add Renaissance or Renaissance Ultra. Use as directed.

Further Resources

- -

Here are just a few titles of books that I have found to be useful and informative.

- -

Natural Facelift by Juliette Kandoo, HarperCollins, 1998. This treatise by a former ballerina contains excellent exercise routines for every muscle of the face and is a good guide to overall facial toning.

Reverse the Aging Process of Your Face: A Simple Technique That Works by Rachel Perry, Avery Publishing, 1995. Ms. Perry presents a process called epidermabrasion (an exfoliation method that can be done at home) and discusses the what and how of skin care.

The Wrinkle Cure by Nicholas Perricone, M.D. Time Warner, 2001. This is the book that started the alternative skin care revolution.

Ko bi do: Japanese Facial Massage by Shogo Mochizuki, Kotobuki Publications, 1999. Exploring facial massage from the Eastern perspective, this very thorough book goes deep into the musculature of the face and describes how to utilize many techniques and modalities not used by Western massage therapists.

Don't Go Near the Cosmetics Counter Without Me by Paula Begoun, Beginning Press, latest revised edition 2003. This classic in the beauty business examines the offerings of virtually every major (and some minor) commercial line of cosmetics and skin care products.

The Yoga Way to Figure and Facial Beauty by Richard Hittleman, Hawthorn Books, Inc, 1968. A great introduction to yoga exercises that anyone (almost) can do.

West Coast Practitioners

Marie-Véronique Nadeau, BA
Licensed aesthetician, antiaging and rosacea consultant

phone: 510-486-9792

toll-free: 1-888-339-9633

Email: *marieveronique@m-vskintherapy.com*

www.organicskintherapy.com

Colette DeVore, LAc, MA Chinese Medicine
Skin Care Specialty: Facial Sculpting (see Chapter Nine)

Devore Acupuncture, Colette Devore

C/O Health Medicine Institute

3799 Mt. Diablo Boulevard

Lafayette, CA 94549

phone: 510-741-7902

email: *colettedevore@devoreacupuncture.com*

www.devoreacupuncture.com

Elke Savala, Certified Ayurvedic Therapist, holistic therapist

Skin Care Specialty: Antiaging and skin rejuvenation from the inside

phone: 510-525-2956

www.Ayurveda-Therapy.com

Dr. Shandor Weiss, ND, Lac
Skin Care Specialty: Dr. Weiss uses a wide variety of therapies including antiaging and natural bio-identical hormone therapy, diet and nutrition, botanical and neutraceutical medicines, homeopathy and flower essences, LED Pulsed Light Therapy, acupuncture and Color Light Acupuncture, allergy and environmental medicine, detoxification, immune therapies, brain balancing, and the best natural and organic skin care products.

Arura Clinic

233 Fourth Street

Ashland, OR 97520

phone: 541-488-1198

www.aruraclinic.com

East Coast Practitioners

Walter Zernis MT, Skin Care Speciality: Massage Therapist Walter Zernis has been practicing for over twenty five years and is a nationally certified massage therapist and bodyworker. He has also done extensive work with athletes at NYC tri-athlete and marathon races. He is currently one of the only practitioners on the East Coast to offer a unique and effective Facial Sculpting technique that manually aligns the muscles of the face to reduce lines and puffiness around the eyes, and lift cheekbones and mouth corners.

39 Clayton Place

Ridgefield, CT 06877

phone: 203-894-1231

www.Quest4health.net

About the Author

Marie-Véronique Nadeau, 58, is a skin-care products formulator and writer. She is CEO and head of product development for Marie-Véronique Skin Therapy, an organic and therapeutic skin-care line. (*Organic* means the products are good for you, *therapeutic* means they actually produce results.)

She became interested in alternative skin care after trying conventional treatments for her rosacea for many years without seeing improvement. Her success with treating rosacea clients led her to think about alternative treatments for skin issues we all inevitably face, at least eventually—namely, wrinkles, sagging, and other signs of aging. Her solutions adhere to the same principles that form the core of her company's philosophy: first, do no harm, and second, do some good. In particular, be good to yourself, and be good to your skin. *The Yoga Facelift* is a vital cornerstone of the dermal do-gooder's credo. Bodily exercise is to liposuction as facial exercise is to Botox and plastic surgery—it doesn't take a rocket scientist to figure out which is better for you in the long run.

The reward for her work is in seeing an M-V face radiating health and beauty, something any one of us can achieve, at any age.

Marie-Véronique has a B.A. in mathematics with a minor in chemistry. Product development (a.k.a. tinkering) is her first love. She also likes reading, writing, cats, emus, and goats—in various descending orders depending on her mood, or theirs. Her daughter Jay L. Nadeau, an honest-to-goodness rocket scientist, assists with laboratory testing and protocol design. She has agreed to collaborate on the second book, which will go into skin-care realms no human has visited before.

Acknowledgments

This book would not have been possible without the unfailing support of my life partner, Wayne L. Silka, as well as so many other friends who comprise a list too long to mention.

To the folks at Red Wheel/Weiser and especially to Elise Collins, who showed me the way, to Brenda Knight, who believed in me, to Maija Tollefson for the gorgeous layout, to Jan Johnson for her expertise, to Caroline Pincus, a fantastic editor, and to Bonnie Hamilton for her knowledge and enthusiasm—my everlasting love and gratitude.

A heartfelt thanks to the models who gave so generously of their time and their FABULOUS faces: Oshala-Dianne Marcus, Amy Nadeau, Angeline Rodriguez-Abeyta, Tanya Henderson, Beth Bachtold, and Claire Cooley.

And a special thanks to Sabrina Marie, my new granddaughter, who chose to pop into the world at about the same time as this book, and who is so good at an exercise we all once excelled at, namely, screaming her head off.

To Our Readers

Conari Press, an imprint of Red Wheel/Weiser, publishes books on topics ranging from spirituality, personal growth, and relationships to women's issues, parenting, and social issues. Our mission is to publish quality books that will make a difference in people's lives—how we feel about ourselves and how we relate to one another. We value integrity, compassion, and receptivity, both in the books we publish and in the way we do business.

Our readers are our most important resource, and we value your input, suggestions, and ideas about what you would like to see published. Please feel free to contact us, to request our latest book catalog, or to be added to our mailing list.

Conari Press

An imprint of Red Wheel/Weiser, LLC

500 Third Street, Suite 230

San Francisco, CA 94107

www.redwheelweiser.com